Venous Access
Made Easy

T0186303

Venous Access Made Easy

James Michael Forsyth
Ahmed Shalan
Andrew Thompson

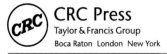

CRC Press
Taylor & Francis Group
Boca Raton London New York

CRC Press is an imprint of the
Taylor & Francis Group, an **informa** business

CRC Press
Taylor & Francis Group
6000 Broken Sound Parkway NW, Suite 300
Boca Raton, FL 33487-2742

© 2019 by Taylor & Francis Group, LLC
CRC Press is an imprint of Taylor & Francis Group, an Informa business

No claim to original U.S. Government works

Printed on acid-free paper

International Standard Book Number-13: 978-1-138-33536-3 (Hardback)
978-1-138-33453-3 (Paperback)

This book contains information obtained from authentic and highly regarded sources. While all reasonable efforts have been made to publish reliable data and information, neither the author[s] nor the publisher can accept any legal responsibility or liability for any errors or omissions that may be made. The publishers wish to make clear that any views or opinions expressed in this book by individual editors, authors or contributors are personal to them and do not necessarily reflect the views/opinions of the publishers. The information or guidance contained in this book is intended for use by medical, scientific or health-care professionals and is provided strictly as a supplement to the medical or other professional's own judgement, their knowledge of the patient's medical history, relevant manufacturer's instructions and the appropriate best practice guidelines. Because of the rapid advances in medical science, any information or advice on dosages, procedures or diagnoses should be independently verified. The reader is strongly urged to consult the relevant national drug formulary and the drug companies' and device or material manufacturers' printed instructions, and their websites, before administering or utilizing any of the drugs, devices or materials mentioned in this book. This book does not indicate whether a particular treatment is appropriate or suitable for a particular individual. Ultimately it is the sole responsibility of the medical professional to make his or her own professional judgements, so as to advise and treat patients appropriately. The authors and publishers have also attempted to trace the copyright holders of all material reproduced in this publication and apologize to copyright holders if permission to publish in this form has not been obtained. If any copyright material has not been acknowledged please write and let us know so we may rectify in any future reprint.

Except as permitted under U.S. Copyright Law, no part of this book may be reprinted, reproduced, transmitted, or utilized in any form by any electronic, mechanical, or other means, now known or hereafter invented, including photocopying, microfilming, and recording, or in any information storage or retrieval system, without written permission from the publishers.

For permission to photocopy or use material electronically from this work, please access www.copyright.com (http://www.copyright.com/) or contact the Copyright Clearance Center, Inc. (CCC), 222 Rosewood Drive, Danvers, MA 01923, 978-750-8400. CCC is a not-for-profit organization that provides licenses and registration for a variety of users. For organizations that have been granted a photocopy license by the CCC, a separate system of payment has been arranged.

Trademark Notice: Product or corporate names may be trademarks or registered trademarks, and are used only for identification and explanation without intent to infringe.

Library of Congress Cataloging-in-Publication Data

Names: Forsyth, James Michael, author. | Shalan, Ahmed, author. |
Thompson, Andrew (Andrew Roger), author.
Title: Venous access made easy / James Michael Forsyth,
Ahmed Shalan, Andrew Thompson.
Description: Boca Raton : CRC Press, 2018.
Identifiers: LCCN 2018048587| ISBN 9781138335363 (hardback : alk. paper) |
ISBN 9781138334533 (pbk. : alk. paper) | ISBN 9780429433801 (ebook)
Subjects: | MESH: Catheterization, Peripheral--methods |
Ultrasonography--methods | Vascular Access Devices | Vascular Surgical
Procedures--methods
Classification: LCC RC78.7.U4 | NLM WB 365 | DDC 616.07/543--dc23
LC record available at https://lccn.loc.gov/2018048587

Visit the Taylor & Francis Web site at
http://www.taylorandfrancis.com

and the CRC Press Web site at
http://www.crcpress.com

I dedicate this book to my wife, Eveline.

With all my love,

James

LIST OF VIDEOS

CONTENTS

INTRODUCTION

Our Collective Experience of Venous Access

As vascular surgery clinicians, we are accustomed to all manners of vascular access. We insert simple cannulas, ultrasound-guided cannulas, midlines, PICC lines, tunnelled catheters and totally implanted ports. We also perform endovenous ablation procedures for the treatment of varicose veins, create arteriovenous fistulas for dialysis access and perform angioplasty procedures for peripheral vascular disease.

Within our own hospital, we specifically provide an 'assisted access' service which centres on midline and PICC line placement. The commonest indications for such lines are long-term intravenous antibiotics, total parenteral nutrition and chemotherapy. We insert hundreds of lines each year, and the demand continues to grow. Indeed, the demand is often much greater than what we as a small number of vascular specialists can easily manage amidst our numerous other specialist commitments. We believe, therefore, that although our training and experience make us ideally placed to provide all forms of vascular access, there is still a need for some of these skills to be taken up by the wider medical and nursing community.

Benefits of 'Assisted Access' Services

Despite the pressure on us to provide such a service, we are acutely aware of its massive benefits, in particular:

- *The service benefits patients.* One definitive and reliable venous line inserted under ultrasound guidance using local anaesthetic for both short- and long-term use is preferable to multiple repeated painful cannulation attempts. Patients receive their infusions on time, meaning that underlying medical conditions are treated promptly. Many patients are also able to go home with their lines for outpatient treatment.
- *The service benefits individual doctors and nurses.* The provision of vascular access varies greatly depending upon the medical institution. However, in our institution, many nurses, specialist nurses and doctors have learned the necessary skills for ultrasound-guided venous access and have benefited tremendously from this. Indeed, the ability to provide assisted access is seen more and more as a necessary skill for the modern healthcare professional.
- *The service is beneficial for the hospital institution.* Our service has led to cost savings, improved governance, improved ward and outpatient

efficiency, and a consolidation of expertise with ultrasound-guided venous access. Being able to discharge patients home for outpatient intravenous therapy has also resulted in reduced bed pressures and improved hospital capacity.

- *The service is beneficial for radiology and anaesthetic departments.* Our service has undoubtedly resulted in a significant reduction in pressure on radiology and anaesthetic departments. As the number of ultrasound-guided cannulas, midlines and PICC lines has increased, the request rates for central lines and tunnelled catheters have plummeted.

Current Issues with Venous Access

Our learning curve throughout the development of our own assisted access service has revealed some areas for improvement:

- *There is a lack of understanding within the medical community about the types of access and indications for use.* Most nurses and doctors understand cannulas and central lines. However, there appears to be widespread confusion as to what midlines, PICC lines, tunnelled catheters and totally implanted ports are.
- *Venous access is approached in a fairly haphazard manner.* The most common approach to venous access we observe is this: cannulate the patient's arm repeatedly; if that doesn't work, cannulate the other arm; if that doesn't work, try the foot; if that doesn't work, call a senior; if the senior is unsuccessful, call for an anaesthetist; and if the anaesthetist cannot insert a cannula, then he/she will insert a central line in theatre. This approach is extremely common, and there does not seem to be much of a sensible thought process behind it (and it is certainly not in the patient's best interest).
- *Ultrasound-guided peripheral venous access is seen predominantly as a 'specialist' skill.* Although we see these procedures as very simple to learn, the general impression we get is that most other doctors/nurses think they are very difficult procedures that demand very high-skill levels. Therefore, most other healthcare professionals avoid learning the technique and simply rely upon the 'specialists'.

Why We Created *Venous Access Made Easy*

This book/video project stemmed from our desire to spread the benefits of such a service to other healthcare professionals and medical institutions around the world. Our vision is to produce a simple and realistic guide to help doctors and nurses make significant improvements in their approach to venous access. We want this guide to make a positive difference for patients, healthcare professionals and healthcare institutions alike. These are our key goals:

1. Enable the provision of and responsibility for high-quality venous access to be moved away from the reduced number of specialists and instead be owned by the far greater number of generalists within the medical and nursing community.
2. Allow more patients to be treated in community and outpatient settings through the use of midlines and PICC lines, thereby reducing inpatient hospital pressure.
3. Adapt and incorporate the most up-to-date techniques and technologies to bring 'vascular access for all' into the twenty-first century.

We hope you find this book and the accompanying videos interesting and inspiring, and above all highly relevant to your daily clinical practice. We created it for everyone: nurses, junior doctors, medical and surgical registrars, emergency medicine doctors, anaesthetists, intensivists, orthopaedic surgeons, cardiologists, and so on. Every doctor and nurse in every hospital in the world can benefit from learning the skills and techniques we describe in this guide.

ACKNOWLEDGMENTS

First and foremost we wish to thank the individual patients who were involved in the production of *Venous Access Made Easy*. It was you, your stories and your real venous access challenges that we hope have given this guide authenticity and credibility.

We also thank the following individuals at York Teaching Hospital (England) who helped make this project possible:

- Susan Chappell, Principal Operating Department Practitioner
- Lucy Clegg, Charity Fundraising Manager
- Nikhil Dhokia, Senior Radiographer
- Susie Dick, Team Manager, Radiography
- Maria Falcone, Theatre Practitioner
- Amanda Forster, Theatre Practitioner
- Liz Hill, Directorate Manager of Surgery
- Matt Smith, Theatre Practitioner
- Donna Sykes, Theatre Practitioner

There were four other parties that were instrumental in the production of this book/video guide. Firstly, we are indebted to Miranda Bromage and Samantha Cook at CRC Press/Taylor & Francis for their patience, commitment, wisdom and guidance. Secondly, we are incredibly grateful to Vygon (UK) Ltd for supporting our vision; in particular we acknowledge the individual contributions of Julie Shepherd, Jason Ram, Linda Kelly and John Thomson. Thirdly, we thank Ballater Medical Ltd (Point of Care Solutions) and Dr John McCafferty for providing us with the cutting-edge wireless ultrasound technology that is bringing venous access into the twenty-first century. Finally, we thank Cal Carey, our videographer and photographer, for his exceptional work and total professionalism. It has been a joy and a blessing working with you all.

ABOUT THE AUTHORS

James Michael Forsyth MBBS MRCS PGDip (HPE) is a vascular and endovascular surgery registrar completing his specialist training in the Yorkshire Deanery, England. He qualified from St George's Hospital Medical School (University of London) in 2011. He has a passion for medical education and service improvement, and also has specific interests in diabetic foot disease and vascular access.

Ahmed Shalan MBBS MRCS ChM is a vascular surgery trainee in the West Midlands, England. He graduated from Cairo Medical School in 2007. He moved to England in 2013, and served as a speciality doctor in vascular and endovascular surgery in York Teaching Hospital for 5 years where he developed and coordinated the assisted venous access service. He has a passion for patient and medical education.

Andrew Thompson MBBS BMedSci MD (Res) FRCS (Gen) is a consultant vascular surgeon and the lead clinician for North Yorkshire Vascular Unit. He qualified from The Royal London and St Bartholomew Hospitals Medical School in 1998, wrote his thesis on abdominal aortic aneurysm genetics at the University College London for the British Heart Foundation in 2007, and completed his training with the Oxford postgraduate deanery in 2010. He spent a year (2011) as the Vascular Society of Great Britain and Ireland Endovascular Fellow at St Mary's Hospital, London. He is currently a consultant vascular and endovascular surgeon at York Teaching Hospital NHS Foundation Trust where he manages all major vascular pathology as part of a team of surgeons and radiologists, for a population of 800,000. His interests include distal reconstruction, renal access, complex abdominal aortic surgery and thoracic outlet syndrome.

PART 1
VENOUS ACCESS PLANNING

CHAPTER 1
VENOUS ACCESS GLOSSARY

Cannulas

Cannulas are short peripheral access devices that are intended for short periods of use, i.e., <96 hours. In adult use, they range in size from the smallest (blue) up to the largest (orange). They are typically inserted via the back of the hand or in the forearm/antecubital fossa. Cannulas can be inserted under direct vision; however, the use of ultrasound is helpful in cases of difficult cannulation (**Figures 1.1** to **1.3**).

Midline

The midline is inserted under ultrasound guidance, traditionally via the upper arm basilic vein. It has to be inserted under strict aseptic conditions. Midlines can be used for both short-term and long-term venous access (i.e., weeks to months). The most common indication for a midline insertion in our unit is

Size	Colour	Flow rate	Uses
14 G	Orange	240 mL/min	Major haemorrhage, rapid large-volume fluid replacement
16 G	Grey	180 mL/min	Trauma, major surgery, GI bleeds, high-fluid volumes
18 G	Green	90 mL/min	Blood products, irritant medications, contrast study
20 G	Pink	60 mL/min	General use, maintenance fluids, IV antibiotics
22 G	Blue	36 mL/min	Small or fragile veins/back of hand

Figure 1.1 Cannula gauges and indications.

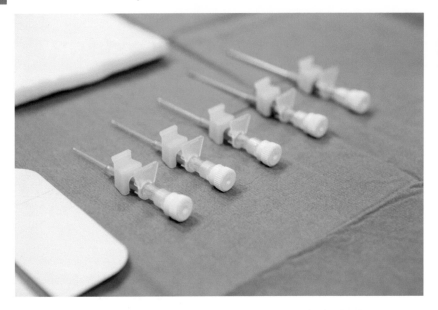

Figure 1.2 Blue and pink cannulas.

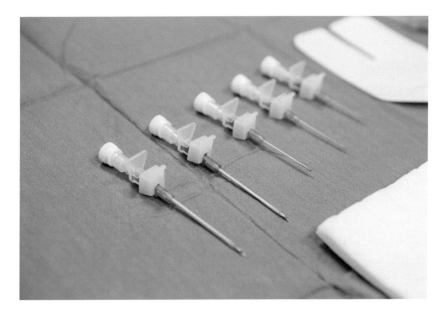

Figure 1.3 Larger cannulas (green, grey and orange).

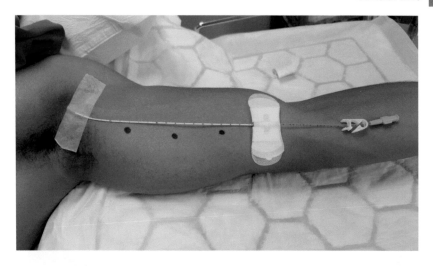

Figure 1.4 Midline with black dots representing the basilic vein marked with ultrasound.

for long-term intravenous antibiotics. However, they can be used for the same indications as a peripheral cannula. If peripheral access is needed for over 4 days, then a midline should be considered instead of repeated peripheral cannula insertions (**Figure 1.4**).

Peripherally Inserted Central Catheter (PICC) Line

The PICC line is of a similar design to a midline. It is inserted in the same way, but because of its extra length, the tip is placed in the central venous system, i.e., in the super vena cava/cavo-atrial junction. It is usually inserted under x-ray or electrocardiogram (ECG) guidance. It is recommended for use in cases when medium-/long-term central access is required, e.g., for chemotherapy, total parenteral nutrition, etc. PICC lines can last up to 12 months or more if they are well cared for (**Figures 1.5** and **1.6**).

Central Line

Central lines are predominantly inserted into the neck via the internal jugular vein. They can also be inserted via the subclavian vein just below the clavicle, or, as a last resort, via the common femoral vein in the groin. They are used when short-term central access is required (<10 days). They come in either single-lumen or multi-lumen forms. They can be used for the administration

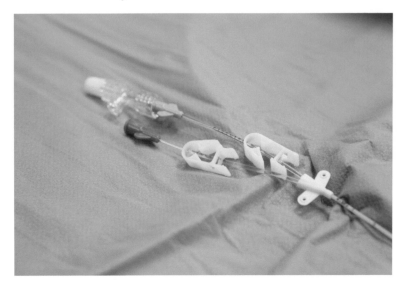

Figure 1.5 Double-lumen PICC line.

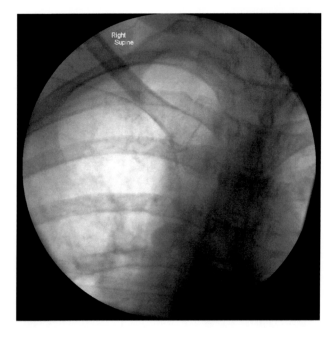

Figure 1.6 Right-sided PICC x-ray confirmation with the tip approaching the cavo-atrial junction.

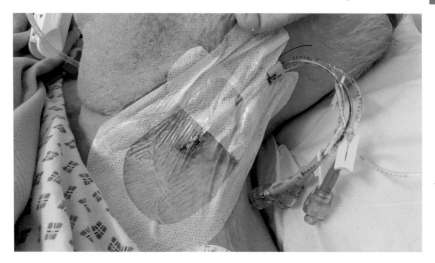

Figure 1.7 Central line – left internal jugular vein (IJV).

of all intravenous solutions, including antibiotics, fluids, medications, parenteral nutrition and chemotherapy. They are excellent for resuscitation and haemodynamic monitoring. Patients having major surgery often have them inserted in theatre (**Figure 1.7**).

Tunnelled Catheter

These lines are used in cases when long-term central access is required. They are inserted via the subclavian or internal jugular veins and the line is tunnelled out onto the skin of the chest wall. The line typically has a cuff that creates a fibrotic reaction under the skin of the chest wall to help seal the line in place (to prevent easy line dislodgement and proximal spread of infection). They are inserted by endovascular specialists and specialist nursing staff in theatre/radiology settings under x-ray guidance. They are usually inserted with the patient awake with local anaesthetic. Such lines can be used for long-term intravenous antibiotics, chemotherapy and total parenteral nutrition. If well cared for, they can last for years (**Figures 1.8** and **1.9**).

Renal Dialysis Catheters

There is a range of temporary and permanent dialysis catheters for use in both acute and chronic renal failure settings. Again, they are inserted via the central veins under ultrasound. Long-term dialysis catheters are tunnelled

7

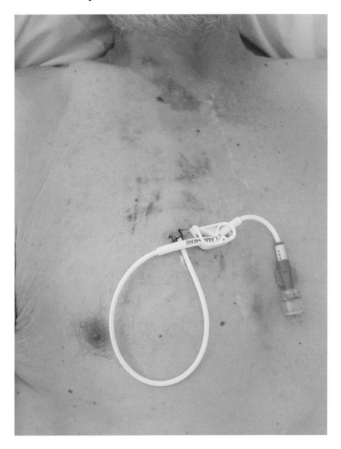

Figure 1.8 Tunnelled catheter for infective endocarditis long-term intravenous antibiotic treatment.

out onto the skin as with the previously mentioned tunnelled catheters. Dialysis patients will often have such a line fitted whilst they are waiting for a more definitive form of vascular access, i.e., fistula/peritoneal dialysis line (**Figures 1.10** and **1.11**).

Totally Implanted Port

These are totally implantable long-term tunnelled central lines. They are most commonly inserted into the subclavian or internal jugular veins and the catheter is tunnelled under the skin of the chest wall. In contrast to

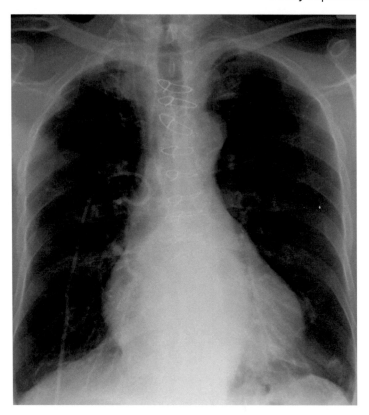

Figure 1.9 Tunnelled catheter – check x-ray.

tunnelled catheters, a surgical cut-down opens up a pocket in the chest wall to allow the port to be inserted there and for the catheter to connect onto it. Once the wound is closed, the port can be accessed by inserting a needle through the skin into the port. They are particularly beneficial for patients requiring chemotherapy who want a discreet venous access option. They require insertion by a vascular and endovascular surgery specialist in theatre with x-ray screening. The patient will usually require a general anaesthetic, although a local anaesthetic approach is still possible (**Figures 1.12** to **1.14**). Such ports can also be inserted through the superior vena cava system via catheterization of the axillary vein, or via superficial veins like the external jugular, cephalic and basilic veins. Exceptionally, the femoral or great saphenous veins can also serve as access points when there is thrombosis of the superior vena cava system.

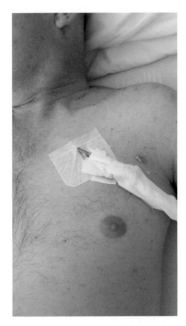

Figure 1.10 Long-term dialysis line.

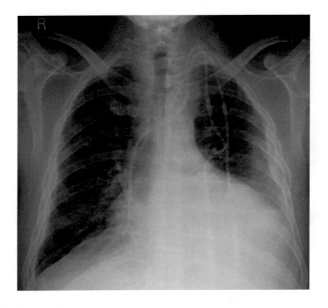

Figure 1.11 Dialysis line – check x-ray.

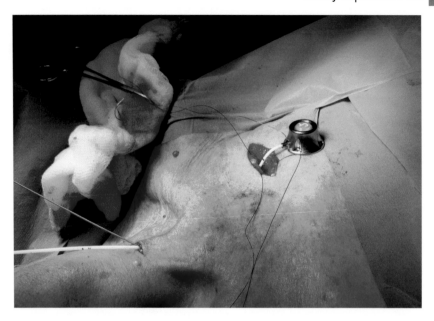

Figure 1.12 Port visible before it is secured in place to chest wall beneath skin.

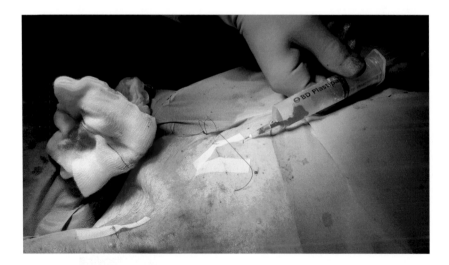

Figure 1.13 Port implantation operation complete with non-coring needle and syringe being used to aspirate and flush the line.

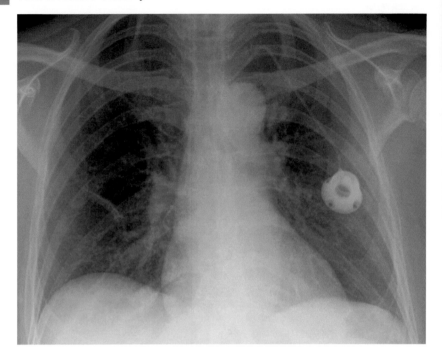

Figure 1.14 Left internal jugular vein totally implanted port – check x-ray showing line tip positioned in lower third of superior vena cava.

CHAPTER 2

VENOUS ANATOMY

RELEVANT VIDEO: https://youtu.be/VDVRhaWVRkA

Video 1 describes the relevant upper limb arteriovenous surface anatomy that should be watched in conjunction with reading this chapter.

Dorsal Venous Arch (Veins on Back of Hand)

The dorsal venous arch lies on the central aspect of the dorsum of the hand. It receives tributaries from the dorsal metacarpal veins. The medial end of the arch forms the basilic vein, whilst the lateral end forms the cephalic vein. This venous arch shows great anatomical variation. The veins on the back of the hand are the most common site for peripheral venous cannulation (**Figure 2.1**).

Cephalic Vein

It begins as a continuation of the lateral end of the dorsal venous arch. It travels across the lateral aspect of the forearm to reach the anterior aspect of the cubital fossa, where it gives rise to the median cubital vein. It then ascends on the lateral aspect of the biceps muscle. The cephalic vein stays superficial to the fascia until it pierces the clavi-pectoral fascia at the level of the delto-pectoral groove. Here it joins the axillary vein. Of note, the cephalic vein is smaller than the basilic vein and may be tortuous as it as ascends the upper arm. Due to the small diameter and potentially tortuous path, the risk of insertion-related phlebitis and thrombosis is increased with this approach; therefore, this vein is not the first choice for midline or PICC line placement.

13

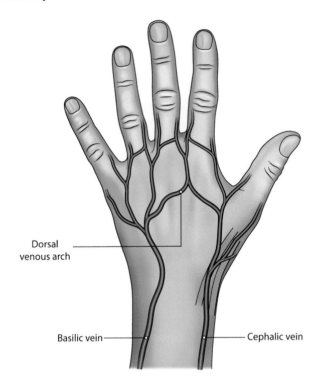

Dorsal
venous arch

Basilic vein ———————— Cephalic vein

Figure 2.1 Diagram showing the anatomy of the dorsal venous arch.

Median Cubital Vein

It arises from the cephalic vein at the lower aspect of the cubital fossa. It passes upwards and medially to join the basilic vein just above the level of elbow. It lies superficial to the bicipital aponeurosis, which separates the vein from both the median nerve and the brachial artery underneath. It is a common site for venepuncture or peripheral venous cannulation because the vein is often superficial, prominent and easily palpable. This site is particularly relevant in unstable patients who require immediate large-bore venous access. It is not a vein recommended for midline or PICC insertion due to it being in an area of flexion, which is known to potentially lead to mechanical phlebitis.

Basilic Vein

It begins as a continuation of the medial end of the dorsal venous arch. It then ascends along the medial aspect of the forearm until it reaches the elbow to receive the median cubital vein. It then runs along the medial aspect of the biceps muscle and dives deep to the fascia in the middle of the arm. The basilic vein above the elbow is the optimal vein of choice for midline and PICC line placement due to the fact that it is the largest of the three upper arm veins and provides a straight and direct route towards the central venous system.

Brachial Vein

The brachial vein is a deep vein in the arm; this vessel is paired closely with the brachial artery and median nerve. The brachial vein carries the highest risk of damage to adjacent structures and should therefore only be accessed with ultrasound guidance and advanced operator experience.

Axillary Vein

The basilic and brachial veins join to form the axillary vein. The axillary vein is joined by the cephalic vein to form the subclavian vein around the level of the clavicle.

Central Veins

The axillary vein continues behind the clavicle as the subclavian vein. It is joined by the jugular veins and curves down behind the sternum to become the brachiocephalic vein. Both brachiocephalic veins join up to form the superior vena cava, which then enters into the right atrium of the heart. Of note, the cavo-atrial junction (which is where PICC line tips are ideally placed) corresponds to the level of the third/fourth intercostal space (**Figure 2.2**).

Lower Limb Venous Anatomy

Great Saphenous and Femoral Veins

The great saphenous vein begins on the medial aspect of the dorsum of the foot. It runs in front of the medial malleolus, then along the medial aspect of the leg a hand's-breadth behind the medial aspect of the patella. It ends by joining the femoral vein at the sapheno-femoral junction 4 cm below and lateral to the pubic tubercle.

The most common site to access the great saphenous vein is at the ankle level in front of the medial malleolus. Subcutaneous cannulation or venous cutdown is possible here, and this is particularly relevant in cases of

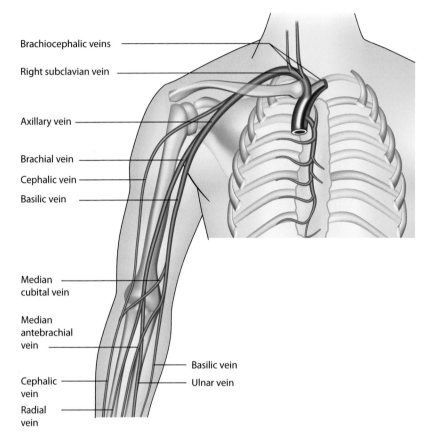

Figure 2.2 Upper limb and central veins.

haemorrhagic shock, as will be described later. The great saphenous vein is also cannulated in cases of endovenous ablation for varicose veins.

Short Saphenous and Popliteal Veins

The short saphenous vein begins on the lateral aspect of the dorsum of the foot, courses around and behind the lateral malleolus, and runs upwards along the middle aspect of the posterior leg. It ends in the popliteal fossa at the back of the knee by joining the popliteal vein.

It is very uncommon to use the short saphenous vein for venous access. It is, however, of particular relevance for endovenous ablation for patients with varicose veins secondary to short saphenous vein reflux (**Figure 2.3**).

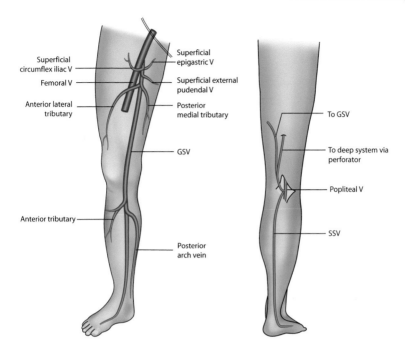

Figure 2.3 Great saphenous vein (GSV), short saphenous vein (SSV), popliteal and femoral veins.

Neck Venous Anatomy

External Jugular Vein

It begins below and behind the angle of the mandible (within or below the parotid gland). It is formed by the union of the posterior auricular and posterior branch of the retro-mandibular veins. It runs vertically across the sternomastoid muscle. It goes deep to the fascia above the level of the clavicle. It ends in the subclavian vein behind the middle of the clavicle.

Internal Jugular Vein

The internal jugular vein is formed by the joining of blood from the sigmoid sinus of the dura mater and the common facial vein. The internal jugular vein runs with the common carotid artery and vagus nerve inside the carotid sheath. The vein, artery and nerve lie underneath the sternomastoid muscle, which runs from the mastoid process behind the ear down towards the sternum. It provides venous drainage for the contents of the skull. This is one of the commonest veins used for central access (**Figure 2.4**).

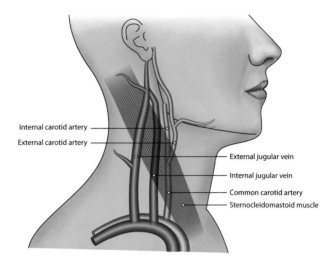

Internal carotid artery

External carotid artery

External jugular vein

Internal jugular vein

Common carotid artery

Sternocleidomastoid muscle

Figure 2.4 External and internal jugular veins.

CHAPTER 3

BASIC ULTRASOUND USE

RELEVANT VIDEO: https://youtu.be/t2cuKWVEo_g

Video 2 describes a basic ultrasound assessment of the upper limb and central veins that should be watched in conjunction with this chapter.

What Is Ultrasound?

Ultrasound is an imaging technique that uses high-frequency sound waves and their echoes. It is similar to SONAR used by submarines.

In ultrasound, the following occurs:

1. The ultrasound machine transmits high-frequency sound pulses into the body via a transducer probe.
2. The sound waves travel into the body and hit the boundaries between the tissues, i.e., between fluid and soft tissue, soft tissue and bone.
3. Some of the sound waves are reflected backwards towards the probe, whilst some travel further on until they reach another boundary and get reflected.
4. The reflected waves are picked up by the probe and relayed back to the ultrasound machine.
5. The machine calculates the distance from the probe to the tissue or organ using the speed of sound in tissue and the time of each echo's return.
6. The machine displays the distances and intensities of the echoes on the screen, forming a two-dimensional image.

The Ultrasound Machine

Ultrasound machines come in various shapes and sizes. However, they will all share the same basic components:

- Transducer probe – Probe that sends and receives the sound waves
- Central processing unit (CPU)
- Transducer pulse controls – Changes the amplitude, frequency and duration of the pulses emitted from the transducer probe
- Display – Displays the image from the ultrasound data processed by the CPU
- Keyboard/cursor – Inputs data and takes measurements from the display

The transducer probe is the main part of the ultrasound machine. It produces the sound waves and receives their echoes. The transducer probe generates and receives sound waves using a principle called the piezoelectric effect. In the probe there are quartz crystals called piezoelectric crystals, and when an electric current is applied to these crystals, they vibrate rapidly. The vibrations produce sound waves that travel outwards. Conversely, when sound or pressure waves hit the crystals, they emit electric currents. Therefore, the same crystals can be used to send and receive sound waves (**Figure 3.1**).

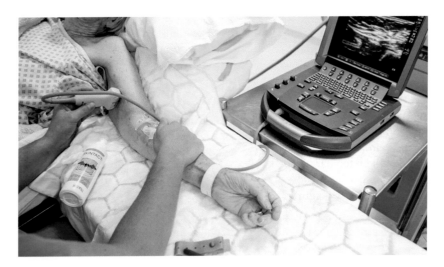

Figure 3.1 Portable ultrasound machine being used to scan arm prior to PICC line insertion.

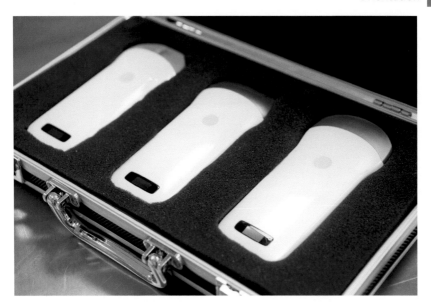

Figure 3.2 Different wireless ultrasound probes of varying frequencies. The blue ultrasound probe has the highest frequency and is most suitable for venous cannulation.

Frequency

It is important to use the highest-frequency probe that reaches the depth required. In the context of upper limb venous access, the veins are usually fairly superficial; therefore, a high-frequency probe is better (**Figure 3.2**).

Gain

The gain control improves the vision on the ultrasound screen. It is similar to the brightness control. It should be manipulated to optimise the image of the vein prior to the procedure. If the gain is too low, the entirety of the image will be too dark; and vice versa; if the gain is too high, the whole image will be too bright. Choose a setting that enables you to identify the relevant structures clearly (**Figure 3.3**).

Orientation

Most ultrasound machines have markers to allow correct orientation. This is often in the form of a groove on one side of the transducer probe which corresponds to an orientation marker on the ultrasound screen. Another simple

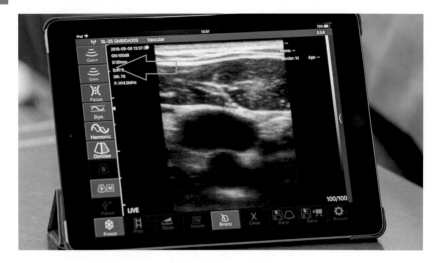

Figure 3.3 Gain up and down buttons on a tablet screen.

way to confirm correct orientation is to touch one side of the transducer with your finger, and if it is correctly oriented, there should be a flicker on the same side of the screen.

Transverse Orientation

In this orientation, the vessel will appear round. If a puncture is performed in the centre of the probe, this will lead to a puncture in the centre of the vessel.

Longitudinal Orientation

In this approach, the vessel will be displayed as a black structure running across the screen. When puncturing the vessel and inserting the guidewire/sheath in this orientation, you will be able to see them passing along the line of the vein for some distance (**Figures 3.4** and **3.5**).

Blood Vessel Characteristics on Ultrasound

It is important to be able to recognise what is an artery and what is a vein. In the context of midlines and PICC lines, it is most important to be able to identify the basilic vein, brachial vein and brachial artery (**Figure 3.6**).

Twenty-First Century Ultrasound

Modern technology has given birth to the wireless ultrasound probe that can be connected to a smartphone or tablet. These wireless ultrasound probes are

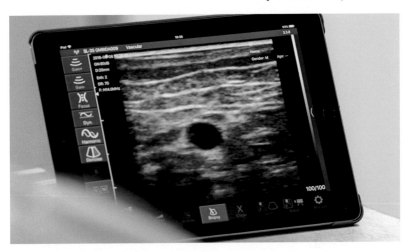

Figure 3.4 Transverse orientation vein.

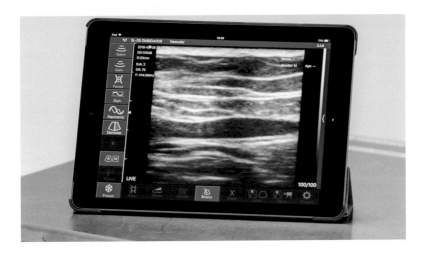

Figure 3.5 Longitudinal orientation vein.

	VEIN	ARTERY
APPEARANCE	Black	Black
MOVEMENT	None	Pulsatile
COMPRESSIBILITY	Yes	No (unless compress very hard)
SIZE	Usually larger than artery	Usually smaller/rounder than vein

Figure 3.6 Ultrasound characteristics of arteries and veins.

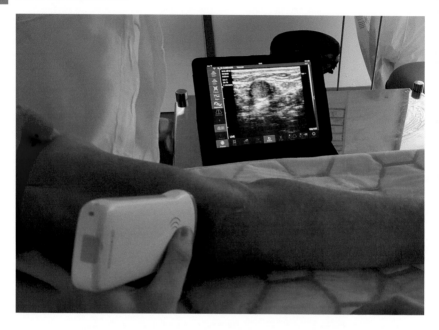

Figure 3.7 Wireless ultrasound probe and tablet visualising the basilic vein in upper medial arm.

smaller, cheaper, simpler and arguably more 'practical' for their role in assisted venous access (**Figure 3.7**).

There are various wireless ultrasound probes and downloadable wireless ultrasound applications available. We recommend carefully reading the individual manufacturer's instructions for use. However, these are the most relevant practice points:

- Ensure you have the B-mode ultrasound setting selected.
- Choose the 'vascular' image setting.
- With the application we use (see **Video 2**), you can adjust the depth of the image by sweeping the screen up or down with your finger. For venous access, you will likely require the most superficial image possible.
- To alter the overall brightness of the image, you can increase or decrease the gain by pressing the increase or decrease button on the screen display.
- To measure the size of vessels, you will first have to freeze the image and then drag the measuring pointers to each side of the vein (**Figure 3.8**).

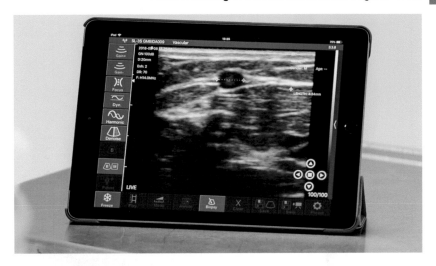

Figure 3.8 Measuring a vein on ultrasound.

Basic Upper Limb Venous Ultrasound Assessment

Once you have made sense of the ultrasound application, you should practise scanning your own arm (or a colleague's) to get a feel for how it works. We recommend putting a tourniquet reasonably tight around the upper arm (axillary level) so that the arm veins will be engorged and easy to identify. As the ultrasound waves must travel through a medium, you will need to apply some ultrasound gel to your arm and/or the ultrasound probe (**Figure 3.9**).

Now you can run the ultrasound probe up and down the arm, identifying suitable veins for cannulation. You can judge whether the veins are suitable for cannulation by compressing them and determining their size and position. A vein that will not easily compress is likely occluded. The most ideal veins for cannulation are large, compressible and away from major neurovascular structures, and have as straight a path as possible. This is why for midlines/ PICC lines, the basilic vein is often ideal (**Figure 3.10**).

Neck Scanning to Assess the Internal Jugular Veins

If there are no suitable veins in either arm for cannulation, then the ultrasound can be used to scan the internal jugular veins in the neck (for consideration of central venous access). In this situation, ask the patient to turn his/her

25

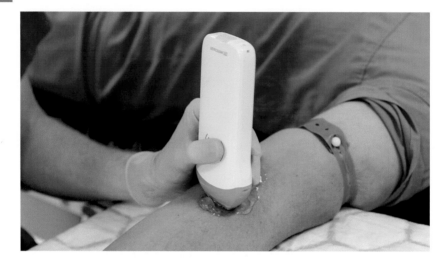

Figure 3.9 Ultrasound probe scanning a patient's arm with gel applied.

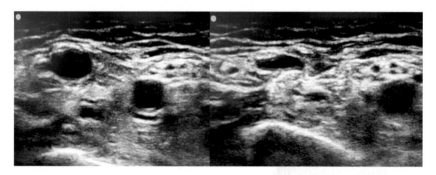

Figure 3.10 Ultrasound images of a basilic vein and brachial artery. The image on the right shows the basilic vein is easily compressible over the humerus bone whilst the artery is not.

head to the opposite side to expose the sternocleidomastoid muscle running down from the mastoid process behind the ear towards the sternal head of the clavicular bone. This is where the internal jugular vein and carotid arteries are positioned (deep to the muscle). Place the probe over this part of the neck in transverse or longitudinal position and adjust the depth to optimise your view. Again, assess the suitability of the internal jugular vein by checking its compressibility (**Figures 3.11** to **3.13**).

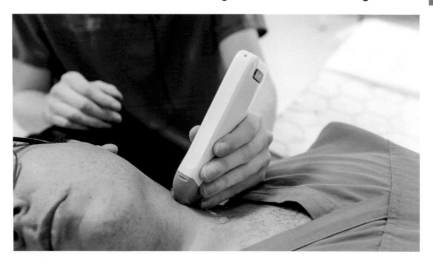

Figure 3.11 Neck being scanned.

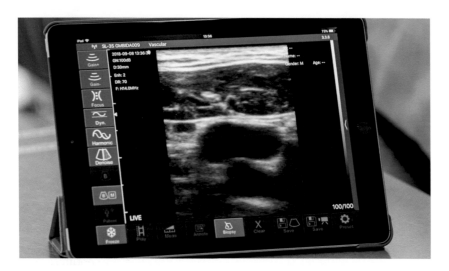

Figure 3.12 Internal jugular vein and carotid artery lying underneath the sternocleidomastoid muscle.

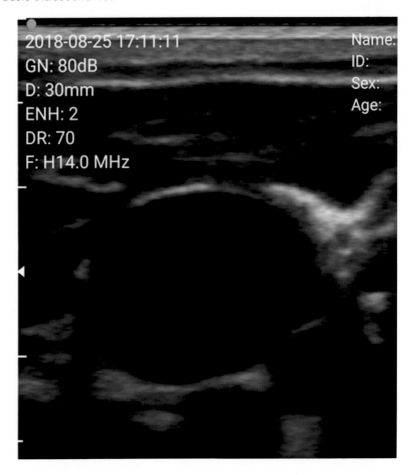

Figure 3.13 Internal jugular vein and both internal and external carotid arteries.

Common Mistakes to Avoid with Ultrasound-Guided Venous Access

- Focusing too much on your hands and the needle, instead of focusing on the ultrasound screen.
- Holding the ultrasound probe incorrectly.
- Too much pressure with ultrasound probe, which collapses the vein.
- Puncturing at the wrong angle.
- Not keeping the vessel of interest in the centre of the screen.
- Not inserting the needle at the centre point of the ultrasound probe.
- Being in an uncomfortable position.

CHAPTER 4

VENOUS ACCESS ASSESSMENT

The venous access assessment should not take you more than 10 minutes to complete. It is designed to help optimise your approach to venous access. It is primarily a clinical assessment that is supported by a simple ultrasound assessment and a review of the patient-specific records. For straightforward patients, the full assessment is probably excessive. However, for patients with challenging venous access, the full assessment is recommended.

Determine the Indication for Venous Access

Patients will require venous access for different reasons and for different lengths of time. The indications will fall broadly into the following categories:

- Intravenous antibiotics
- Intravenous medications/fluids/blood products
- Total parenteral nutrition
- Chemotherapy
- Radiology investigations requiring intravenous contrast, e.g., computed tomography (CT) scanning
- Dialysis access

There may be various degrees of overlap between these indications. The choice of venous access approach must therefore be flexible, and should be tailored towards the patient's individual needs.

Focused History

- **What is the patient's preferred choice of access?**
  A patient may be right-handed and want to do crosswords whilst in hospital, and therefore would prefer you to target the left arm, or vice versa. In an ideal world, try to use the side the patient prefers.

- **Have there been prior venous access issues?**
  For example, patients may tell you that their veins are very difficult to identify and doctors/nurses always struggle to cannulate their veins. In this context, an ultrasound-guided approach should be considered.

- **Previous venous access procedures?**
  Patients may have had previous midlines, PICC lines or central/tunnelled lines. Pacemakers, renal dialysis lines and renal access fistulas should also be considered under this heading. Such procedures can distort normal anatomy and lead to venous scarring/fibrosis/thrombosis.

- **Previous upper limb/central vein deep vein thrombosis (DVT)?**
  As an example, a patient with a previous left arm DVT which resulted in axillary vein thrombosis may lead to difficulty with midline/PICC line access from this side, which should prompt you to try the right side instead.

- **Any relevant upper limb or neck trauma/radiotherapy/surgery?**
  Such factors may have led to central vein compression, scarring or fibrosis. This could result in central vein stenosis or obstruction. This could create significant challenges with venous access.

- **Any risk factors for bleeding or venous thrombosis?**
  Patients on antiplatelet agents or anticoagulants will obviously have an increased bleeding risk. For peripheral access, this is rarely a major issue, but for central access and tunnelled/implanted lines, this will be of greater significance. Likewise, patients with risk factors for venous thromboembolism will be at a greater risk of a DVT/pulmonary embolism (PE).

- **Do future venous access requirements need to be considered?**
  For example, a patient with worsening chronic renal failure may be under consideration for an arm fistula in the near future. In such a context, you should ideally avoid cannulating the cephalic vein at the wrist or in the antecubital fossa in the non-dominant arm.

Focused Examination

- *Visual inspection of the entire upper limbs, neck and chest wall.*
  An inspection of these areas will give you a clear visual indication of the most appropriate form of access. It may also highlight potential problems with access. For example, a sign of central venous stenosis/obstruction includes a swollen arm/neck/face with collateral veins visible around the upper chest wall.

- *Specific examination of the veins in upper limbs (+/− tourniquet).*
  Patiently and thoroughly exploring the upper limbs for suitable veins is highly recommended. Don't rush in at the first vein you see; there may be a more suitable alternative that is better for the patient. If veins are not immediately apparent, you can use warm water, gravity and a tourniquet to make veins easier to identify. This should allow the veins to fill up more, hopefully making cannulation easier.

Bedside Ultrasound Assessment

- An ultrasound can be an incredibly helpful tool at your disposal. A handheld wireless ultrasound that can connect to a smartphone or tablet is ideal. A simple ultrasound assessment of the patient's upper limb venous circulation and central venous system should take you less than a minute.

Review the Patient-Specific Records

- *Look at the drug chart.* Are there any medications that could create problems, e.g., anticoagulants?
- *Look at the observation chart.* Is the patient stable or unstable?
- *Review the blood results.* If the patient's platelet count is extremely low, do you need haematology advice? If the patient's inflammatory markers are completely normal, are you sure they need a line for intravenous antibiotics?
- *Look at any relevant radiology imaging.* For example, a chest x-ray may show a pacemaker on the left, indicating potential issues for a left-sided PICC placement. An enormous fungating upper chest or neck cancer visible on CT scan might involve the central venous system, meaning central access could be extremely challenging or dangerous.

CHAPTER 5
CHOOSING THE RIGHT VENOUS ACCESS APPROACH

In this chapter, we will review some realistic and challenging case examples that will show you how to apply the venous access assessment in 'real-world' settings. We start with simple cases and work upwards to more complex scenarios. To begin with, we provide you with an overview of the venous access options available and the contexts in which they are applicable. Of note, the primary purpose of this guide is to help you develop the skills to insert cannulas, ultrasound-guided cannulas and midlines/PICC lines. In our opinion, these represent the foundation of the 'triangle' of venous access (**Figure 5.1**).

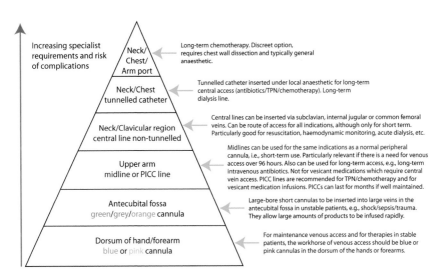

Figure 5.1 The 'triangle' of venous access.

CASE 1

A 94-year-old male patient with multiple comorbidities admitted with severe community-acquired pneumonia and acute kidney injury. Background of multiple recent long hospital admissions for falls and urinary tract infections. Has scanty visible or palpable veins in both his hands and forearms, which are heavily bruised from multiple previous cannulation attempts (**Figure 5.2**). Ultrasound assessment reveals normal central veins and healthy basilic and cephalic veins in the upper arm and forearms.

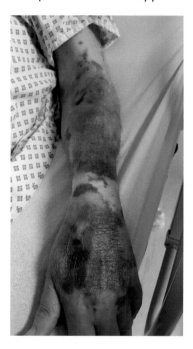

Figure 5.2 Patient with very bruised arm following multiple venous access attempts.

The likelihood is that this patient will be a hospital inpatient for at least a week, if not longer. The severe pneumonia and renal failure secondary to sepsis and dehydration will probably require multiple days of venous access for intravenous antibiotics and fluids. With relatively poor peripheral venous access for cannulas, and the likely requirement for repeated cannulation attempts, it is sensible to consider a midline in this patient.

Correct choice = MIDLINE

CASE 2

A 38-year-old otherwise fit and well female patient admitted with lower limb cellulitis that has not improved despite 3 days of oral antibiotics at home. The patient is systemically well, and her inflammatory markers are only mildly raised. She has excellent venous access via back of hands and both forearms (large veins easily visualised and palpable even without use of a tourniquet) (**Figure 5.3**).

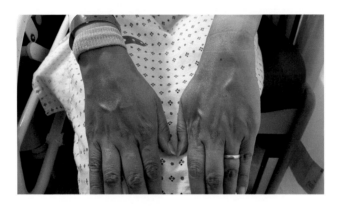

Figure 5.3 Good veins on back of hands.

This woman is likely to require only a few days of intravenous antibiotics to settle down the cellulitis, and will almost certainly be discharged from the hospital very soon. Given her excellent venous supply, she would be most suitable for a normal blue or pink cannula in the dorsum of the hand. She would not require an ultrasound assessment.

Correct choice = BLUE/PINK CANNULA

CASE 3

A 70-year-old woman, one year after a total hip replacement. Two months ago, she had removal of a cement remnant which was causing chronic hip pain. Unfortunately, this has been further complicated by a deep wound infection that requires 6 weeks of intravenous antibiotics. The patient had a left-sided midline inserted the week before, but this line got infected and had to be removed. The orthopaedic team has requested another

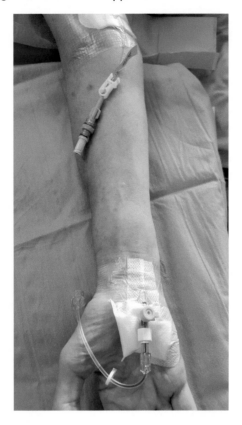

Figure 5.4 Midline in right arm with pink cannula sited in wrist with proximal swelling and erythema.

midline. Her left upper arm is swollen and tender. The right arm has bruises in the forearm and antecubital fossa, and there is a pink cannula inserted in the volar aspect of the wrist which is causing pain and swelling. Ultrasound assessment reveals a decent basilic vein in the right upper arm.

This woman's left arm would not be suitable for a repeat midline on the left given that it is swollen and tender. The right arm would therefore be the next option. Of note, as can be seen in the picture above, the woman has been cannulated numerous times already on the right arm, and the pink cannula in the wrist is a very painful site for cannulation. In such a case, a midline should be inserted sooner rather than later in order to spare such patients from multiple painful cannulation attempts (**Figure 5.4**).

Correct choice = RIGHT ARM MIDLINE

CASE 4

A 53-year-old female patient who requires at least 2 weeks of intravenous antibiotics for a complicated urinary tract infection. The medical team looking after the patient is struggling with cannulation. She has no obvious forearm or hand veins on inspection and palpation (despite using a tourniquet). She also has multiple self-harm scars over her forearms which make identifying veins more difficult. At the moment, she has a very fragile pink cannula in the back of her hand which has been bandaged for security. Ultrasound assessment reveals very small veins in her forearms that would be difficult to cannulate, but reasonably sized basilic veins bilaterally.

This woman's forearms/hands are clearly not ideal for cannulation, and as one can observe in the image below, the antecubital fossa veins have already been targeted and left bruised. In this setting, the best option appears to be a basilic vein midline (**Figure 5.5**).

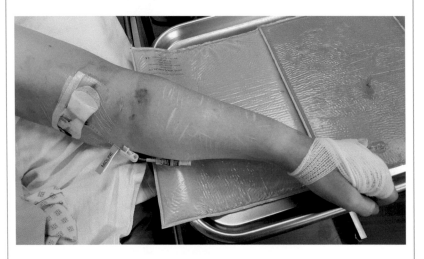

Figure 5.5 Midline in scarred and bruised arm.

Correct choice = MIDLINE

CASE 5

A 49-year-old alcoholic man is admitted onto the acute medical unit with coffee-ground vomiting and bleeding per rectum. He has a systolic blood pressure of 90 mmHg with a heart rate of 110. He is pale, cool, clammy and peripherally shut down. His capillary refill time is 6 seconds. There are 4 bowls of coffee-ground vomit lying beside him. He has clinical signs of chronic liver disease. He also has severe psoriasis, making identification of veins in his forearms difficult.

This patient likely has underlying oesophageal varices due to portal hypertension from chronic liver disease, and is having a large upper gastrointestinal (GI) bleed. He needs immediate large-bore venous access. Orange/grey/green cannulas should be inserted into both antecubital fossae (**Figure 5.6**).

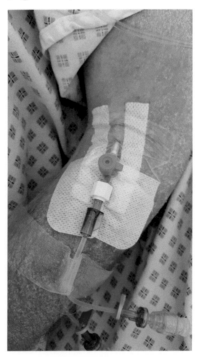

Figure 5.6 Green cannula in antecubital fossa of patient having major upper GI bleed.

Correct choice = GREEN CANNULA

CASE 6

A 50-year-old patient on the orthopaedic ward who has had a surgical washout and revision of an infected total hip replacement (**Figure 5.7**). According to microbiology advice, he will require 6 weeks of intravenous antibiotics. The patient has previously had midlines in his left arm and is adamantly refusing another one because it has caused him chronic upper arm pain. Ultrasound assessment at the bedside reveals normal internal jugular veins on both sides and normal basilic/brachial veins on both sides.

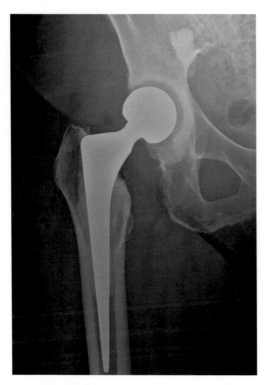

Figure 5.7 Infected total hip replacement.

In this case, a midline would be possible in either arm, but the patient is adamant he does not want one. Given the suitability of the internal jugular veins, the patient would be suitable for a Tunnelled catheter.

Correct choice = TUNNELLED CATHETER

CASE 7

A 65-year-old gentleman admitted to the emergency department with sudden-onset abdominal and back pain with collapse. He has a pulsatile expansile abdominal mass. Heart rate is 110, blood pressure is 80/60 mmHg. The patient is pale, extremely anxious and peripherally shut down. He is awake and communicative with a Glasgow Coma Scale (GCS) score of 15. CT scan reveals a ruptured 10-cm abdominal aortic aneurysm (AAA) (**Figure 5.8**).

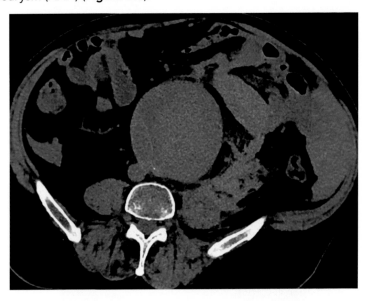

Figure 5.8 Ruptured abdominal aortic aneurysm.

This patient is going to require a lot of blood products, intravenous fluids and intravenous antibiotics in a very short space of time. Getting the patient to theatre as soon as possible is the priority. He needs 2 large-bore cannulas inserted in both antecubital fossae whilst in the emergency department, and then needs to be taken up to theatre straight away. Virtually all patients with a ruptured AAA will have a central line inserted via the neck, but this should be performed in theatre by an anaesthetist after the patient has been put to sleep and the emergency operation has already commenced.

Correct choice = ORANGE/GREY CANNULA + CENTRAL LINE

CASE 8

A 70-year-old gentleman is referred to the acute medical unit with nausea, lethargy, confusion and shortness of breath. These symptoms have come on gradually over the past few months and progressively worsened. The patient's community doctor took some blood the previous day, which has shown that he has a creatinine of 1000, a glomerular filtration of 11 and a potassium of 7.5. The patient has not seen a doctor in years and is not known to a nephrologist. The patient's ECG shows tall T waves and QRS complex slurring. His chest x-ray shows pulmonary oedema. His arms and legs are oedematous, and you cannot easily identify any upper limb veins despite using a tourniquet. Ultrasound assessment reveals good basilic and brachial veins in both upper arms and normal internal jugular veins.

This represents a 'crash' presentation of end-stage renal disease. As can be seen, the patient requires emergency medical treatment for uraemia, hyperkalaemia and pulmonary oedema/fluid overload. Peripheral venous access is clearly challenging, given the limb oedema. You could attempt ultrasound-guided peripheral access to institute treatment for hyperkalaemia and fluid overload. However, what this patient definitively needs is an urgent referral to the renal team for dialysis via a centrally placed line. A short-term dialysis line via a central vein (internal jugular or common femoral veins are commonly used) would be the standard approach (**Figure 5.9**).

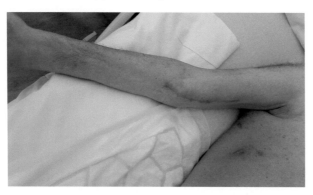

Figure 5.9 Arm of patient with chronic renal failure. A scar on the upper arm from a failed basilic vein transposition fistula can be seen. Renal failure patients, like this patient, have notoriously difficult venous access.

Correct choice = DIALYSIS LINE

CASE 9

An unkempt 29-year-old male is rushed into the emergency department by paramedics with an armed police escort. The patient is violent and aggressive. One of the paramedics is pressing down onto a wound situated on the left side of his neck, which is soaked with bright red blood. The patient also has a partially amputated right arm at the level of the elbow. There is a tourniquet above his elbow which was put on by the paramedics. You get a handover from the paramedic team, who inform you that this gentleman is an intravenous drug user and gang member who is currently under the influence of narcotics (likely cocaine). They also inform you that he is homeless and lives on the streets. Apparently, he got into a knife fight with another gang member who cut the left side of his throat and hacked at his right arm with a machete. There is major arterial bleeding coming from his neck and arm which has currently been controlled with direct pressure on the neck and the arm tourniquet. The patient is thrashing around and pushing you away as you try to assess him.

This patient has two major vascular injuries that are imminently life-threatening. He needs urgent vascular surgery intervention and will go straight to theatre. However, he also represents a case of very difficult venous access. The partial amputation of the right arm means venous access is not possible on this side. The left side is theoretically possible, but he will not keep his arm still and because of his previous drug abuse,

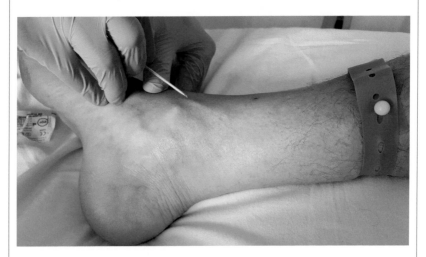

Figure 5.10 Great saphenous vein cannulation above medial malleolus.

he has very poor veins for cannulation. A central line via the neck will not be possible because this is the area where the surgeons are going to be operating. In such a difficult and dire situation, one would have to look at the patient's legs for venous access; that is, try to cannulate the long saphenous vein at the ankle or insert a femoral line via the groin (**Figure 5.10**).

Correct choice = LARGE BORE CANNULA AT ANKLE LEVEL +/− FEMORAL LINE +/− INTRAOSSEUS ACCESS

CASE 10

A 55-year-old female with Crohn's disease and short bowel syndrome on home total parenteral nutrition (TPN) is currently on the cardiology ward for mitral valve endocarditis which will require 6 weeks of intravenous antibiotics. She has had numerous previous central lines, tunnelled catheters and PICC lines on both sides. On this admission, she had a right subclavian vein central line inserted which was complicated by a right-sided pneumothorax for which she has a chest drain *in situ*. She has had the current subclavian line in for 11 days and requires ongoing central access for TPN and intravenous antibiotics. The patient informs you she is right-handed and would prefer the left side to be used for access. Her left arm is not swollen and there are no obvious signs of central venous stenosis or obstruction. Ultrasound assessment reveals a compressible left basilic vein which appears suitable for a PICC line insertion (**Figures 5.11 to 5.13**).

The photographs clearly demonstrate how many venous access procedures this patient has had. On the right side of her neck, you can see multiple scars from internal jugular vein central lines. On her chest wall, she has further visible scars from tunnelled catheter exit sites. The chest drain indicates that the subclavian vein cannulation had directly punctured the pleura, causing a pneumothorax. If a PICC line is required, then the left side would be preferred given the fact that most of the recent interventions have been on the right side (and the patient is right-handed). However, anticipate that the PICC line insertion from the left side may be challenging if she has underlying central vein pathology related to the multiple previous central lines. In such a case, you should insert the PICC line with x-ray/fluoroscopic guidance and consider interventional radiology assistance (venogram images might be needed).

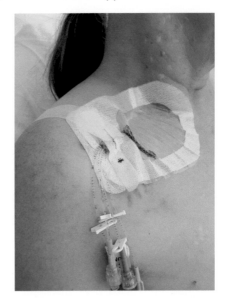

Figure 5.11 Right-side subclavian line with multiple scars on right side of neck from numerous central/tunnelled lines.

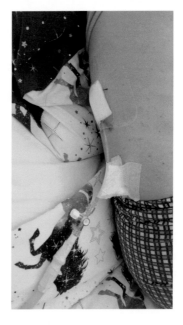

Figure 5.12 Chest drain, right side of chest.

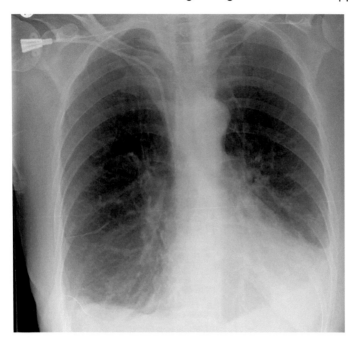

Figure 5.13 Chest x-ray showing right-side subclavian central line *in situ*, along with chest drain and small residual apical pneumothorax.

Correct choice = PICC LINE (LEFT SIDE)

CASE 11

A 58-year-old intravenous drug abuser is admitted with a swollen and infected left groin. On CT scan, there is a 4-cm pseudoaneurysm of the distal common femoral artery. The patient goes to theatre and requires ligation of his femoral artery. Postoperatively, he requires a prolonged course of intravenous antibiotics. His arms are extensively damaged from repeated drug abuse using infected needles. Ultrasound scanning reveals occluded left basilic, brachial and cephalic veins. The right basilic and cephalic veins are patent on ultrasound, although slightly small. His internal jugular veins are both patent and easily compressible (**Figures 5.14** and **5.15**).

This patient has destroyed virtually all of the veins in his hands and forearms. As he requires long-term intravenous access for antibiotics, a midline would be ideal. This could be attempted from the right-hand side. If a midline were not possible, then a tunnelled catheter should be considered.

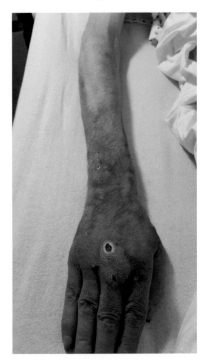

Figure 5.14 Arm of intravenous drug user.

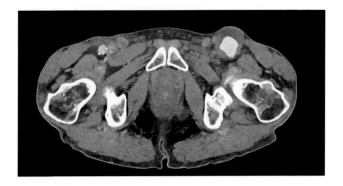

Figure 5.15 Groin pseudoaneurysm on CT.

Correct choice = MIDLINE RIGHT SIDE

PART 2
VENOUS ACCESS PROCEDURES

RELEVANT VIDEO: https://youtu.be/Jc-e8n93zEE

Video 3 demonstrates the peripheral venous cannulation technique that should be watched in conjunction with this chapter.

Our approach for all venous access procedures in this guide revolves around the **4 Ps**:

- Planning
- Preparation
- Positioning
- Procedure

1. Planning
   - Brief clinical assessment.
   - Choose an appropriate site for venepuncture.
   - Choose appropriate cannula depending upon indication for use (**Figure 6.1**).

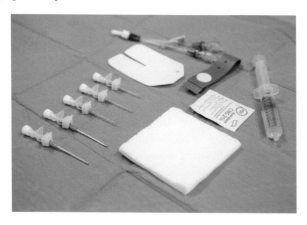

Figure 6.1 Cannula setup with all cannulas to choose from.

2. Preparation
   - Verbal consent and explanation of procedure to patient.
   - Equipment needed (cannula, extension tubing, alcohol wipe, gauze swabs, normal saline flush, tourniquet, cannula dressing).
   - Wash hands and put on non-sterile gloves (you should use a non-touch technique, as a full surgical aseptic technique is not indicated for peripheral cannulation).
   - Prime cannula extension tubing with normal saline.
3. Positioning
   - Make yourself comfortable (use a chair/stool if needed).
   - Make sure the patient is comfortable and his/her arm is resting on a cushioned surface.
   - Position arm according to the vein you intend to cannulate. The dorsal aspect of the hand and forearm are the primary sites we recommend for peripheral cannulation. The antecubital fossa is also recommended for when short large-bore venous access is required. Generally speaking, the flexor aspect of the forearm should be avoided, as this area is sensitive and painful for patients, and the major arteries (radial and ulnar) run along the flexor aspect of the forearm and wrist.
4. Procedure (**ABCDEF**)
   - *Antiseptic.* Standard ANTT approach (Aseptic Non Touch Technique). Use an alcohol wipe to cleanse the area where you intend to cannulate the vein. Allow the alcohol solution time to work and dry (wait for 30 seconds; this will allow the antiseptic to work, and during this time you can communicate to the patient what the rest of the procedural steps are, etc.) (**Figure 6.2**).
   - *Banding.* Apply a tourniquet of moderate tightness proximal to where you intend to cannulate the vein.
   - *Cannula.* Once the vein is engorged and easy to identify, then insert the cannula tip (bevel up) into the vein. Approach the vein at an angle of around 10–20 degrees along the path of the vein. Think of the cannula entering the vein according to the same principles of an airplane touching down on an airport runway (**Figure 6.3**).
   - *Drainage.* Once the cannula has entered the vein, there should be a flashback of venous blood visible at the end of the cannula. At this point, the outer tubing can be fully advanced over the inner needle into the vein, whilst simultaneously withdrawing the inner needle so it is completely removed. After this, blood can be withdrawn from the cannula into blood bottles for laboratory analysis (**Figure 6.4**).
   - *Examination.* Once you have completed the drainage section, you need to confirm that the cannula will function properly. Release the tourniquet and attach the extension tubing. Use your 10-mL

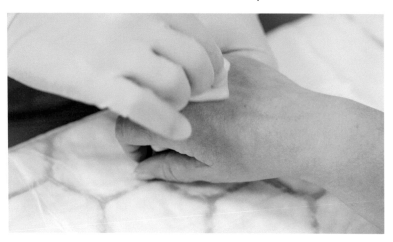

Figure 6.2 Alcohol wipe to dorsum of hand.

normal saline flush to run the fluid through the cannula into the vein. If you encounter resistance, the tissue around the cannula starts to expand and/or the patient experiences pain, then clearly the cannula is not positioned satisfactorily (**Figure 6.5**).

- *Fixation*. Clean the area around where you have cannulated using another alcohol wipe. Use a gauze swab to dry this area afterwards. Once the skin around the cannula is clean and dry, then apply cannulate fixation sticker (**Figure 6.6**).

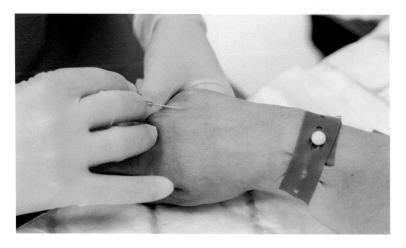

Figure 6.3 Cannula about to puncture vein.

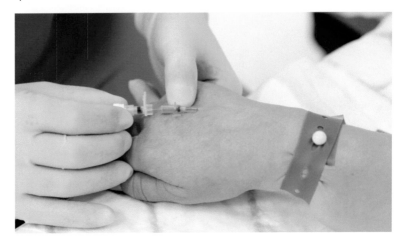

Figure 6.4 Flashback visible in cannula and inner needle being withdrawn.

In closing, you should attach a label to the cannula dressing site with the date of insertion clearly indicated, fill in any required insertion documentation for the patient notes, and dispose of any sharps and clinical waste. Also, thank the patient, make sure he/she is okay, and answer any questions the patient may have.

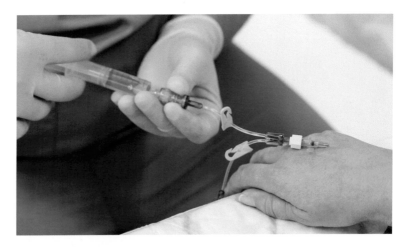

Figure 6.5 Flushing cannula with normal saline.

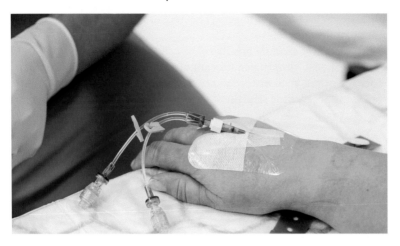

Figure 6.6 Cannula secured in place.

Tips & Tricks for 'Difficult' Venous Cannulation

- Use a tourniquet and be patient. Take your time and explore both upper limbs for a suitable vein.
- By hanging the arms down, gravity can help the veins to fill up and become more prominent.
- Bathing the hands/forearms in warm water (or using a towel soaked in warm water) may help the veins vasodilate and become more prominent.
- Hydrate the patient. If a patient is dehydrated and intravascularly depleted, then it will be more difficult to identify veins. If the oral route is available, then asking the patient to drink a jug of water 1 hour before you attempt cannulation may make the upper limb veins more prominent.
- For patients with upper limb oedema, you can press over the area where you anatomically suspect to find a suitable vein (for around 15 seconds). This will disperse the oedema away from the area of interest and should make it easier to find the vein.
- If you can feel a vein, but cannot easily see it, then you can use a marker pen to identify the palpable borders of the vein, which should help you when inserting the cannula.
- Sometimes the cephalic vein at the wrist is mobile from side to side, which can make cannulation difficult. Therefore, you can use your left index finger and thumb to immobilise the vein as you are aiming to

puncture it close to your fingers. This technique can also be used for other mobile veins.

- Use the smallest cannula possible.
- If it is clear that 'simple' venous cannulation is not possible, despite the above measures, then instead of repeatedly needling the patient to no avail, consider moving straight to an ultrasound-guided approach.

CHAPTER 7

ULTRASOUND-GUIDED PERIPHERAL VENOUS CANNULATION

RELEVANT VIDEO: https://youtu.be/10-JoCNyeNo

Video 4 demonstrates the ultrasound-guided peripheral venous cannulation technique that should be watched in conjunction with this chapter.

If a peripheral venous cannula is indicated, but you cannot confidently see or palpate a vein despite your best efforts, then an ultrasound-guided approach should be considered.

1. Planning
   - Ultrasound assessment of upper limb. With your appreciation of upper limb venous anatomy, using the ultrasound, try to identify a reasonably sized, superficial and sufficiently straight segment of a vein. The cephalic vein in the mid-forearm is usually the best venous access option because it is not commonly used for cannulation, as it is not easily seen by the naked eye. The other recommended choices include the cephalic vein in the upper arm and the basilic vein in the upper medial arm.
   - Choose an appropriately sized cannula depending upon the indication for use.
2. Preparation
   - Verbal consent and explanation of procedure to patient.
   - Equipment needed (ultrasound, non-sterile ultrasound gel, cannula, extension tubing, alcohol wipe, gauze swabs, normal saline flush, tourniquet, cannula dressing) (**Figures 7.1** and **7.2**).
   - Wash hands and put on non-sterile gloves.

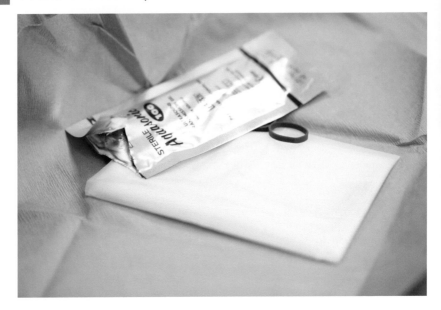

Figure 7.1 Ultrasound gel and sterile ultrasound cover.

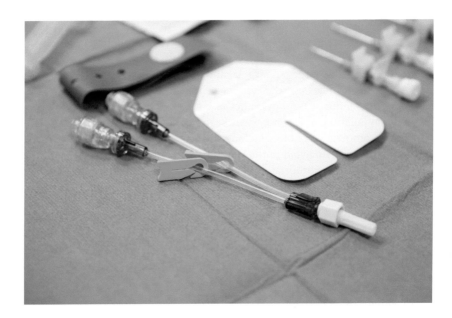

Figure 7.2 Cannula tray setup.

3. Positioning
   - Make yourself comfortable (use a chair/stool if needed). In particular, position the ultrasound screen so that it is directly in front of you so that it is easy to see and you do not have to twist your neck.
   - Make sure the patient is comfortable and his/her arm is resting on a cushioned surface.
   - Position arm according to the vein you intend to cannulate.
4. Procedure (**ABCDEF**)
   - *Antiseptic.* Standard ANTT approach (Aseptic Non Touch Technique). Use an alcohol wipe to cleanse the area where you intend to cannulate the vein of interest. Allow the alcohol solution time to work and dry (wait for 30 seconds; this will allow the antiseptic to work, and during this time you can communicate to the patient what the rest of the procedural steps are, etc.).
   - *Banding.* Apply a tourniquet moderately tightly proximal to where you intend to cannulate the vein.
   - *Cannula.* Apply the non-sterile ultrasound gel above the area where you have already determined you intend to cannulate the vein. With the tourniquet applied, the vein should become engorged and prominent. Position the vein in the centre of the ultrasound screen. Now take a gauze swab and wipe away any residual ultrasound gel below the ultrasound probe where you intend to puncture the skin. Clean this area one more time with an alcohol wipe.

Now take your cannula and insert the tip (bevel up) into the skin around 0.5–1 cm proximal to where the ultrasound probe is positioned, also making sure that the needle enters at the centre point of the ultrasound probe. Have the cannula pointing in the direction of the path of the vein, at an angle between 10 and 30 degrees (**Figure 7.3**).

As you insert the needle, you should see the tip of the needle appear on the ultrasound screen. The tip of the needle should be above the vein. Now move the ultrasound probe backwards a very short distance until the tip of the needle vanishes. Insert the cannula in deeper, and again you will see the tip re-appear on the screen. As you continue this process (called *leading the needle*), you will be able to guide the tip of the needle down to the top wall of the vein of interest. Once the needle has reached the top vein wall as you apply pressure downwards, you will observe the vein wall indent. At this point, apply a small amount of pressure to puncture the vein wall. You should then be able to visualise the tip of the needle within the vein lumen (and if

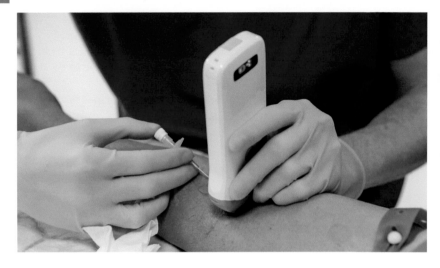

Figure 7.3 Pink cannula advancing into skin under ultrasound guidance.

you are inside the vein, this will be confirmed with a flashback of blood at the end of the cannula) (**Figures 7.4** to **7.6**).

- *Drainage*. At this point, the outer tubing can be fully inserted over the inner needle into the vein, and the inner needle can be withdrawn. At this juncture, blood can be withdrawn from the cannula into blood bottles for laboratory analysis (**Figure 7.7**).
- *Examination*. Once you have completed the drainage section, you need to confirm that the cannula will function properly. Release the tourniquet and attach the extension tubing. Again, use your 10-mL normal saline flush to run the fluid into the vein. You should be able to insert the flush easily into the patient's arm. If you encounter resistance, the tissue around the cannula starts to expand and/or the patient experiences pain, then the cannula is not positioned satisfactorily.
- *Fixation*. Clean the area around where you have cannulated using another alcohol wipe. Use a gauze swab to dry this area afterwards. Once the skin around the cannula is clean and dry, then apply the cannula fixation sticker (**Figure 7.8**).

In closing, you should attach a label to the cannula dressing with the date of insertion, fill in any required insertion documentation for the patient notes, and dispose of any sharps and clinical waste. Also, thank the patient, make sure he/she is okay and answer any questions the patient may have.

LEADING THE NEEDLE TECHNIQUE

Ultrasound guided access approach for peripheral and central vein cannulation

This diagram highlights a mock approach to the left internal jugular vein (e.g. for a central line). The images show a theoretical needle advancing towards the vein through the overlying sternocleidomastoid muscle, with the carotid artery displayed beneath. For peripheral venous cannulation, which is the focus of this chapter, the same approach and principles can be used.

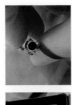
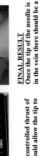
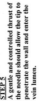
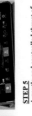
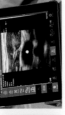
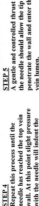
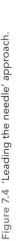
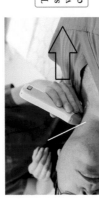

STEP 1
Insert needle (white line) just proximal to ultrasound probe and advance until needle tip first appears on screen (white dot).

STEP 2
Slide probe away from you until the needle tip disappears.

STEP 3
Advance needle further until needle tip reappears.

STEP 4
Repeat this process until the needle has reached the top vein wall. At this point slight pressure with the needle will indent the upper vein wall.

STEP 5
A gentle and controlled thrust of the needle should allow the tip to penetrate the wall and enter the vein lumen.

FINAL RESULT
Once the tip of the needle is in the vein there should be a confirmatory flashback of dark venous blood.

Figure 7.4 'Leading the needle' approach.

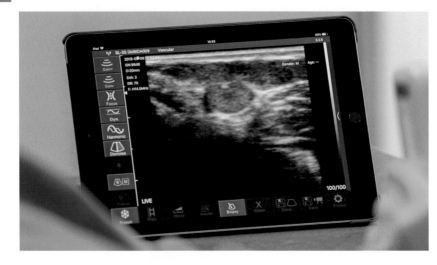

Figure 7.5 Needle tenting at top of vein wall.

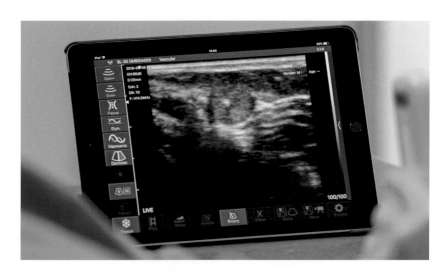

Figure 7.6 Needle inside cephalic vein on ultrasound.

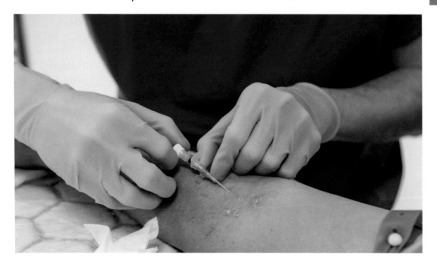

Figure 7.7 Cannula flashback.

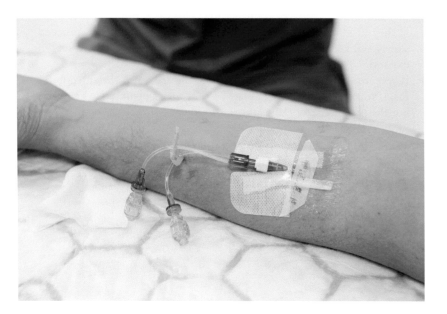

Figure 7.8 Completed ultrasound-guided cannula.

Tips & Tricks for Ultrasound-Guided Venous Cannulation

- Your first attempt at venous cannulation should be at a slightly distal portion of the identified vein. This is so that if your first attempt fails, you will have a healthy section of vein proximal to this for further attempts.
- Take your time. Also, remember to scan both arms to find the most suitable vein.
- Using the ultrasound technique in a transverse section, ensure that you position the vein in the centre of the screen and that you puncture the skin opposite to the centre point of the ultrasound probe. Ensure that the vein and the cannula are in the same plane.
- Make sure that you are able to get the most out of the ultrasound equipment. Become familiar with the basic setup of the ultrasound device and try to optimise the settings so your view is ideal. Also, have the room lighting damped such that there is not excessive light reflecting off the ultrasound screen and obscuring your clarity of vision.
- Ultrasound-guided venous cannulation is a skill that requires both hand-to-hand and hand-to-eye coordination. This takes time to develop and at the outset may be difficult to achieve instantly. Therefore, proceed slowly and keep practising. With greater experience, your skill set will expand.
- If you are scanning the medial aspect of the arm or in the antecubital fossa, you need to ensure that the vessel you are planning to cannulate is not the brachial artery. By applying gentle pressure with the ultrasound probe, venous structures should easily compress, whilst the brachial artery will not easily compress and will clearly be seen pulsating on the screen. Alternatively, you can use colour Doppler if your ultrasound machine has this capability.

CHAPTER 8

MIDLINE INSERTION

RELEVANT VIDEOS: https://youtu.be/YFcxbytYfRc
https://youtu.be/ooLTdBgLPLo

Videos 5 and 6 demonstrate the techniques for a standard and smartmidline™ insertion and should both be watched in conjunction with this chapter.

We describe two particular midlines in this chapter. The smartmidline™ is intended for use in patients who require short-term and mid-term intravenous therapy (up to 29 days). smartmidline™ is a CT rated catheter with the larger gauge sizes (4Fr and 5Fr) being suitable for radiology contrast administration. The 'standard' midline we describe is the Lifecath™ midline, which can be used for the duration of treatment.

Indications

- Intravenous fluid and medication administration suitable for peripheral delivery.
- Delivery of hydrating solutions and nonirritating/isotonic medications.

Contraindications

- Vesicant chemotherapy
- Hyperalimentation fluids
- Mastectomy with lymph node clearance/fistula on ipsilateral side
- Total parenteral nutrition
- Irritating antibiotics

1. Planning
   - Venous access assessment (see Chapter 4).
   - Choose appropriate side for midline insertion.
2. Preparation
   - Written consent obtained from patient.

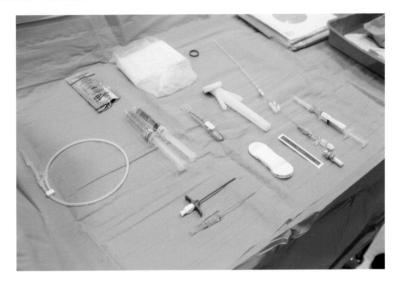

Figure 8.1 Midline equipment tray setup.

- Equipment needed (midline pack, ultrasound machine, sterile ultrasound gel and probe cover, local anaesthetic, cleaning solution for arm, normal saline flushes) (**Figure 8.1**).
- Assistance required → We prefer to have assistance for midline insertion, although single operation is still possible.
- Room setup → The room must be large enough so you do not feel claustrophobic and uncomfortable. There needs to be a bed/ trolley for the patient to lie down on, and an arm board to allow the patient to abduct his/her arm at 90 degrees. You will need a trolley for your sterile midline tray and another trolley/table to position the ultrasound monitor on. You will also require a chair or stool to sit on.
- Prime all catheter lumen with normal saline.

3. Positioning
   - Make yourself comfortable.
   - Make sure the patient is comfortable and his/her arm is resting on a cushioned surface.
   - Position the arm outwards at 90 degrees (abducted and externally rotated position) to give you the best access to the basilic vein.
   - Position the ultrasound screen so it is in front of you (behind patient's abducted arm) (**Figure 8.2**).

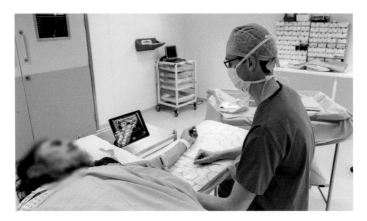

Figure 8.2 Operator sitting down about to do midline with patient's arm abducted at 90 degrees, and ultrasound directly in front of vision.

4. Procedure (**ABCDEF**)

- *Asepsis.* An aseptic technique and surgical scrub is required for all medium- to long-term venous access device insertions. This includes the use of a gown and sterile gloves – surgical ANTT. The upper medial aspect of the patient's arm will need to be cleaned with an appropriate antiseptic solution, and then sterile surgical drapes will have to be placed around the area of interest. The ultrasound probe will also need to be placed into a sterile ultrasound bag with ultrasound gel applied at its tip (**Figures 8.3** to **8.5**).

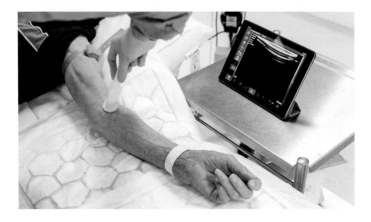

Figure 8.3 Patient's arm being cleaned with alcohol solution.

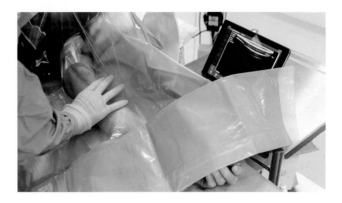

Figure 8.4 Patient's arm being draped.

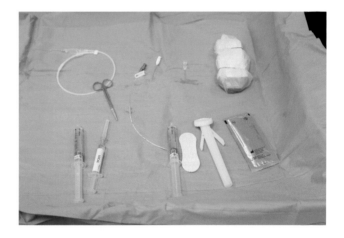

Figure 8.5 Sterile smartmidline™ tray.

- *Banding.* A tourniquet should have been applied at moderate tightness around the upper arm at the axillary level.
- *Catheter.* Use the ultrasound to visualise the basilic vein. It is recommended to puncture at around the centre point of the upper medial arm. Infiltrate the local anaesthetic into the skin where you intend to cannulate the vein. Allow the anaesthetic to take effect (few seconds). Now insert the needle into the skin where you have injected the local anaesthetic. Puncture the vein along the same principles as described in Chapter 7 (i.e., leading the needle) (**Figures 8.6** to **8.9**).

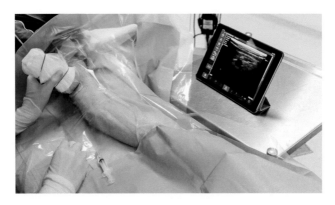

Figure 8.6 Visualising basilic vein on ultrasound just prior to starting procedure.

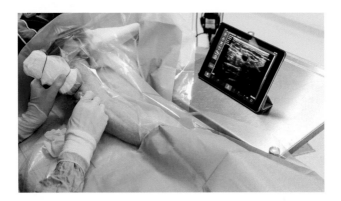

Figure 8.7 Injecting local anaesthetic.

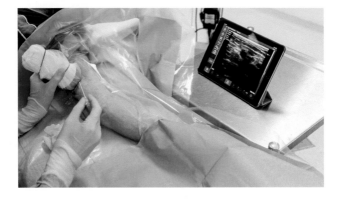

Figure 8.8 Pointing needle into skin below ultrasound.

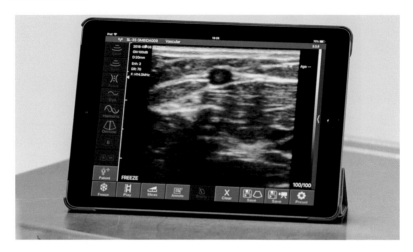

Figure 8.9 Needle in centre of vein on ultrasound.

Once you have punctured the basilic vein, you should place the ultrasound probe safely down beside you and stabilise the needle with your left hand. Now feed the floppy end of the guidewire into the needle and onwards into the basilic vein. We recommend inserting the guidewire into the vein such that you have about half the length of guidewire left outside the patient. At this point, leave the guidewire in place and remove the needle. You can also release the tourniquet at this point (**Figures 8.10** and **8.11**).

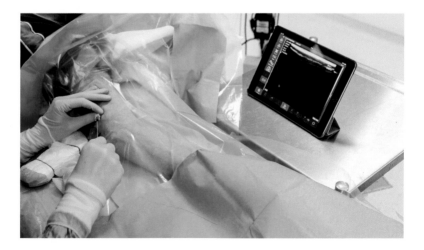

Figure 8.10 Feeding guidewire into needle.

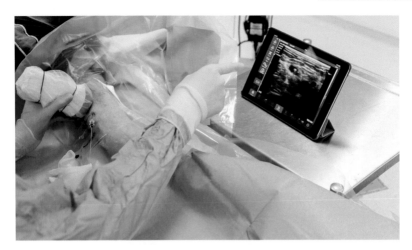

Figure 8.11 Guidewire and needle positioned inside the vein on ultrasound.

Now you are in a position where you have confident access into the basilic vein. For the insertion of a smartmidline™ at this point, you should insert the blue dilator over the guidewire into the patient's arm to open up a tract to allow the midline to be inserted. After removing the dilator, you can then gently feed the smartmidline™ over the guidewire into the vein. Once the smartmidline™ is inside the patient's arm, the inner guidewire can be removed (**Figures 8.12** to **8.13**).

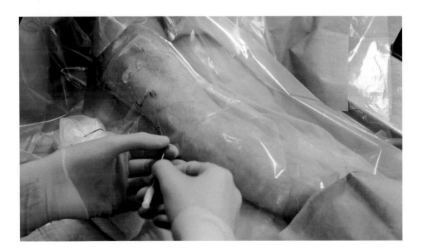

Figure 8.12 Dilator being fed into arm.

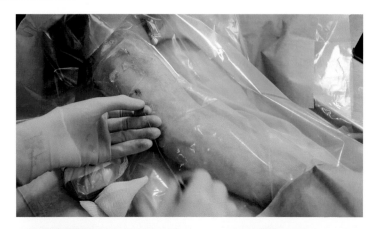

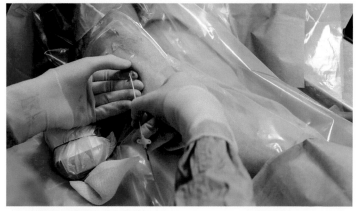

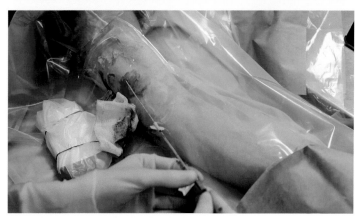

Figure 8.13 smartmidline™ being advanced into arm.

Unlike with a smartmidline™, for a standard midline insertion, a breakable sheath mechanism is used to allow you to insert the midline into the vein. Once the guidewire is inside the vein, you can make a tiny nick in the skin using the blade provided. This will allow you to advance the sheath over the guidewire into the vein. Once the sheath has been inserted into the vein, you can remove the guidewire and inner sheath. There will be a flashback of dark venous blood from the end of the sheath, and at this point you should use your finger to cover this hole and prevent excessive blood loss (you can also place a gauze swab here to collect blood). Now insert the midline fully inside the basilic vein through the outer sheath. With the midline inside the basilic vein, the final step is to snap the outer sheath and separate it. The two sides of the outer sheath will peel away from each other, leaving only the midline *in situ* (**Figures 8.14** to **8.21**).

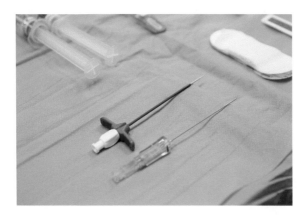

Figure 8.14 Midline sheath used to enable standard midline access to vein.

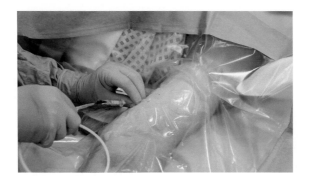

Figure 8.15 Guidewire being advanced through needle into basilic vein.

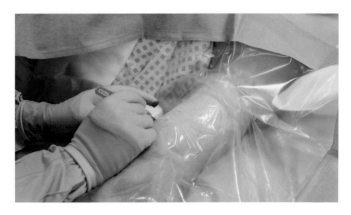

Figure 8.16 Blade used to make a nick in skin to allow sheath to penetrate with ease.

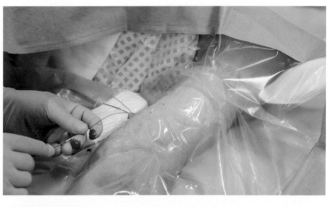

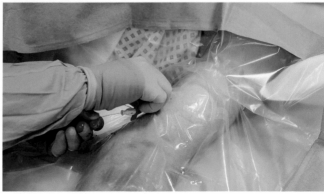

Figure 8.17 Sheath advancing over guidewire into basilic vein.

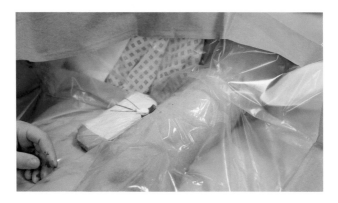

Figure 8.18 Sheath fully inside vein.

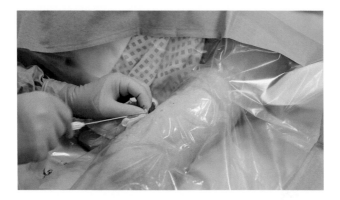

Figure 8.19 Removing inner sheath/dilator and guidewire.

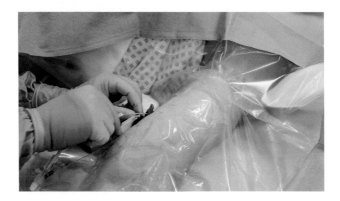

Figure 8.20 Inserting midline through outer sheath.

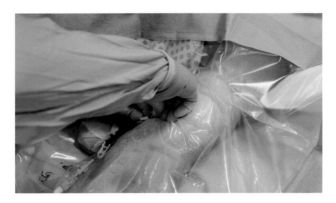

Figure 8.21 Snapping outer sheath to leave only midline *in situ*.

- **Drainage**. Now that the midline is in its final position within the basilic vein, you can remove the inner stylet. Attach the normal saline syringe to the end of the midline and freely aspirate venous blood to confirm it is in the vein.
- *Examination*. Once you have completed the drainage section, you need to confirm that the midline will function properly. Use your 10-mL normal saline flush to run the fluid into the midline. Use a push pause/positive pressure technique. If this can be easily performed and the patient experiences no discomfort, you can be confident that the midline is in a satisfactory position (**Figure 8.22**).

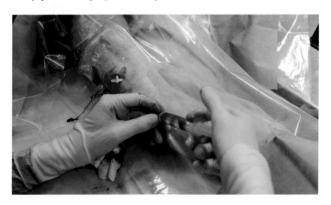

Figure 8.22 Flushing midline with 10-mL normal saline syringe.

- *Fixation*. Using a sterile swab, clean and dry the area around where you have inserted the midline. Apply the fixation device to the midline and then onto the patient's arm (**Figures 8.23** and **8.24**).

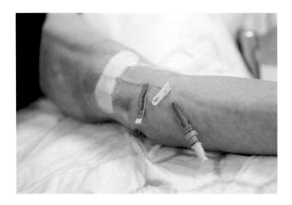

Figure 8.23 smartmidline™ final result.

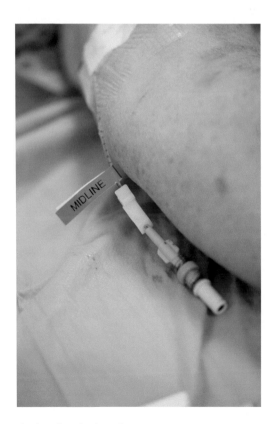

Figure 8.24 Standard midline final result.

In closing, you should label the midline, fill in the insertion documentation for the patient notes, and clear the trolley and dispose of any sharps and clinical waste. Also, thank the patient, make sure he/she is okay and answer any questions the patient may have.

Tips & Tricks for Midline Insertion

- Midline insertion is very straightforward if the vein puncture is successful the first time. However, the chosen vein can go into spasm and haematoma can collect if the first puncture is unsuccessful. Therefore, try to cannulate the vein distally enough so that you still have enough healthy vein proximal to the first puncture site if you require further attempts.
- If the basilic vein is not suitable, then the brachial vein can be considered. However, the brachial vein runs very close to the brachial artery and the median nerve; therefore, you should only attempt to cannulate this vein if you are experienced and you can confidently avoid these other important structures. Otherwise, you should consider the basilic vein on the contralateral arm or try a different venous access approach.
- If whilst you are inserting the midline you encounter resistance, you should scan the vein using the ultrasound to ensure you are indeed inside the vein. If this is the case, then you can flush the midline whilst inserting it → this flushing should expand the vein walls and hopefully will allow the midline to advance.

CHAPTER 9
PICC LINE INSERTION

RELEVANT VIDEO: https://youtu.be/WtliFTeWUPM

Video 7 demonstrates the technique for PICC line insertion using both x-ray and ECG guidance technology and should be watched in conjunction with this chapter.

PICC lines are about 50–60 cm long and are intended to reach the lower superior vena cava/upper right atrium. The ideal final PICC line tip position is the cavo-atrial junction. They are used for the administration of many different types of treatments, but the main difference from midlines is that they allow infusions to be given that are only suitable for central vein administration. They are ideal for patients who require mid- to long-term therapy. The PICC line we describe in this section is the Lifecath™ PICC. There are other types of PICC line available, for example, the Maxflo® Expert PICC, which allows high-pressure injections (particularly good for radiology contrast injections like CT scanning).

Indications
- Total parenteral nutrition
- Infusions with extreme variations
- Vesicant drugs
- Extended duration of intravenous therapy
- Frequent blood draws required

Contraindications
- Coagulopathy
- Mastectomy with lymph node clearance/fistula on ipsilateral side

  1. Planning
     - Venous access assessment (see Chapter 4).
     - Choose appropriate side for PICC line insertion.

2. Preparation
  - Written consent obtained from patient.
  - Equipment needed (PICC line pack, ultrasound machine, sterile ultrasound gel and probe cover, local anaesthetic, cleaning solution for arm, normal saline flushes).
  - Assistance required → We do recommend having an assistant for PICC line insertion.
  - Room setup → The room must be large enough so you do not feel claustrophobic and uncomfortable. There needs to be a bed/trolley for the patient to lie down on, and an arm board to allow the patient to abduct his/her arm at 90 degrees. You will need a trolley for your sterile PICC line tray, and another trolley/table to position the ultrasound monitor on. You will also require a chair or stool to sit on.
  - PICC line positioning technology → Options include ECG technology, live x-ray screening/fluoroscopy, or a formal post-procedural chest x-ray (**Figures 9.1** to **9.5**).

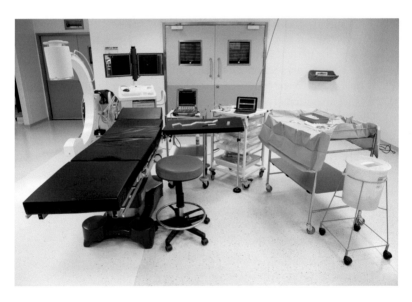

Figure 9.1 Whole room setup with x-ray equipment, ultrasound machine, ECG technology, sterile PICC line tray and trolley with arm board for patient to rest abducted arm on.

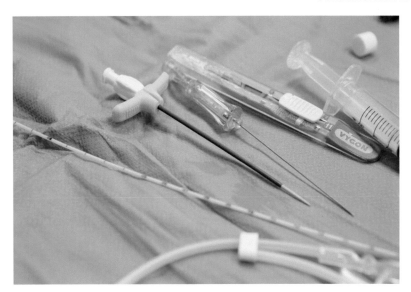

Figure 9.2 Yellow PICC line sheath.

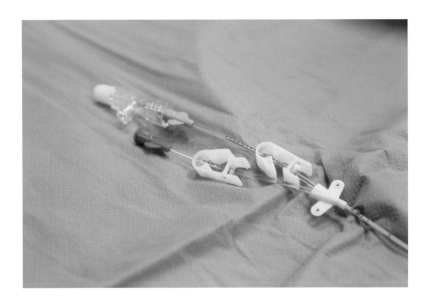

Figure 9.3 Double-lumen PICC line.

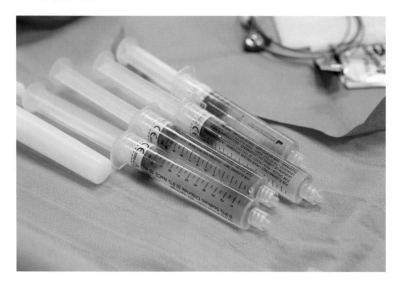

Figure 9.4 4× saline syringes. When using ECG PICC line guidance technology, have plenty of saline syringes to spare, as you use the saline to flush the line to generate an ECG trace.

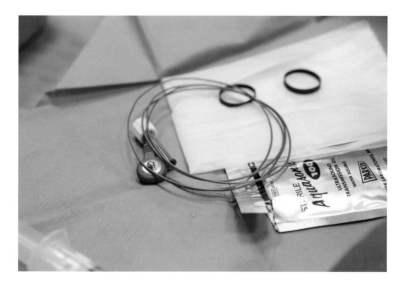

Figure 9.5 Red ECG lead used to connect the end of the PICC line to the ECG machine to generate an intra-cavitary ECG trace.

- Measure the length of the intended PICC line using the tape measure provided. Using the ultrasound, identify a suitable basilic vein in the middle of upper medial arm (left or right). Mark this point on the arm. Measure from this point to the axillary crease, then to the right sterno-clavicular joint (or sternal/jugular notch), then down to the 3rd or 4th intercostal space on the right sternal border. When you are sterile, you can cut the PICC line to this measured length (**Figures 9.6** to **9.8**).
- Prime all catheter lumen with normal saline.

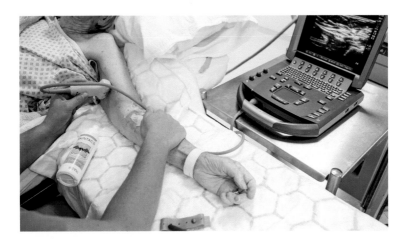

Figure 9.6 Ultrasound scan of arm pre-procedure.

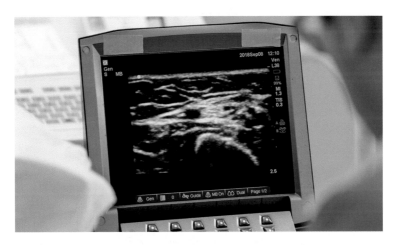

Figure 9.7 Identifying basilic vein for PICC line on ultrasound.

81

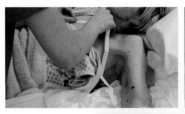
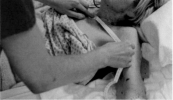
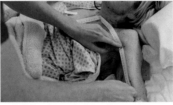

Figure 9.8 Measuring PICC line length using a tape measure.

3. Positioning
   - Make yourself comfortable.
   - Make sure the patient is comfortable and his/her arm is resting on a cushioned surface (**Figure 9.9**).
   - Position the arm outwards at 90 degrees (abducted and externally rotated position) to give you the best access to the basilic vein.

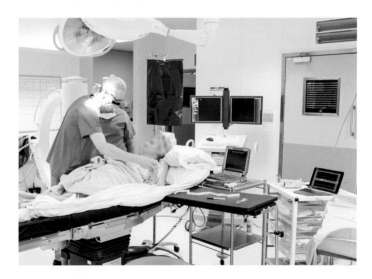

Figure 9.9 Operator introducing himself and comforting patient prior to PICC line insertion.

4. Procedure (**ABCDEF**)

- *Asepsis.* As this is a central venous line, this now specifically requires the use of a sterile gown, gloves, hat and mask – surgical ANTT. The upper medial aspect of the patient's arm will need to be cleaned with an appropriate antiseptic solution, and then sterile surgical drapes will have to be placed around the area of interest. The ultrasound probe will need to be placed into a sterile ultrasound bag with ultrasound gel applied at its tip.
- *Banding.* A tourniquet should have been applied around the upper arm at the axillary level at moderate tightness.
- *Catheter.* Cannulate the vein as per the previous chapter on midline insertion. Once you have reached the point where you have the sheath inserted into the basilic vein, the procedure will be slightly different for a PICC line placement. At this point, the PICC line should have been cut at the intended length as per your previous measurements. To cut the PICC line, you will need to withdraw the stylet back (bend) and cut the catheter using sterile scissors. Re-advance the stylet to the end of the trimmed catheter.

Remove the inner sheath and guidewire and insert the PICC line through the outer sheath into the vein. Insert the PICC line slowly (about 2 cm per second), never forcing it if you encounter resistance. If you do encounter resistance, withdraw the stylet a few centimetres and try to re-advance. As the catheter approaches the patient's shoulder, ask him/her to turn his/her head towards the insertion side and to tuck his/her chin on that shoulder. This will help to avoid cannulating the jugular vein.

If you are using ECG guidance technology, then when you have inserted about 10–15 cm of line, it is time to confirm your ECG connections are in place and that the PICC line is sufficiently flushed with normal saline. As you slowly advance the PICC line, you should periodically pause and check the ECG trace. As the PICC line tip approaches the cavo-atrial junction and sino-atrial node, the P wave should become progressively more positive. Once the P wave has become maximally positive, this represents the tip sitting at the cavo-atrial junction. If you advance the tip further into the right atrium and beyond the sino-atrial node, the P wave will show an increasingly negative deflection. You can therefore use the ECG trace to accurately position the tip of the PICC line (**Figures 9.10** to **9.16**).

If you are using x-ray confirmation for PICC line placement, then you should insert the catheter to the measured length and confirm the final tip position radiologically (**Figure 9.17**).

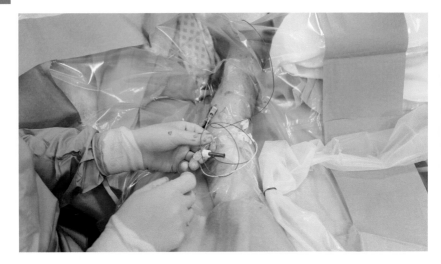

Figure 9.10 Red ECG wire connecting PICC line to ECG machine (which creates the intra-cavitary ECG trace seen on the bottom of ECG screen).

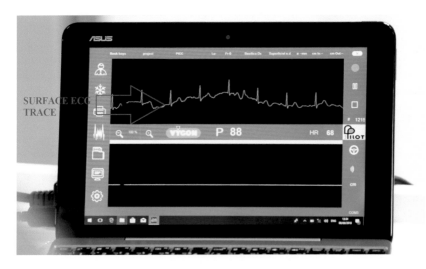

Figure 9.11 Top ECG surface reading showing normal sinus rhythm from the ECG leads which are connected to the patient.

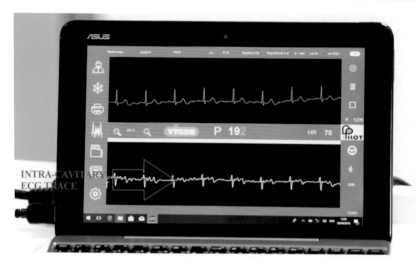

Figure 9.12 Surface and intra-cavitary ECG traces when the PICC line is approaching the heart and the PICC line tip is picking up electrical activity from the sino-atrial node.

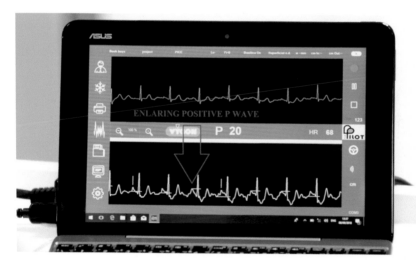

Figure 9.13 There is a clear increase in size of the P wave, indicating that the PICC line tip is progressing down the superior vena cava.

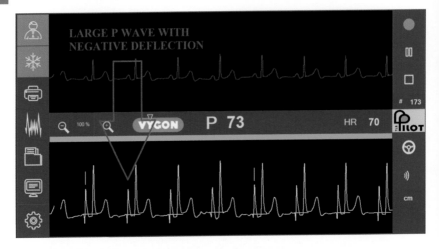

Figure 9.14 The P wave is significantly larger. However, there is a slight negative deflection, indicating that the tip of the line has passed the cavo-atrial junction and is sitting partially in the right atrium.

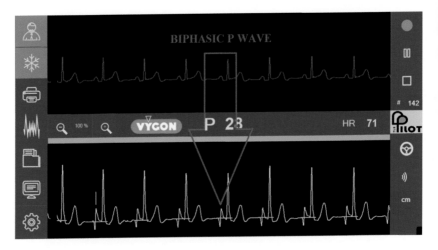

Figure 9.15 P wave is now biphasic, indicating that the tip of the line is now wholly inside the right atrium.

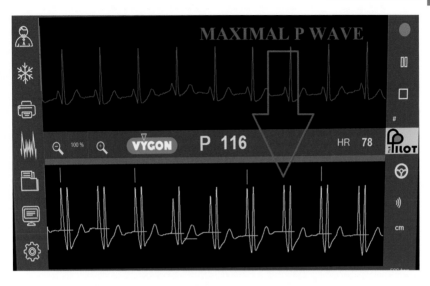

Figure 9.16 Withdrawing the PICC line back to the level of the cavo-atrial junction will produce a maximally positive P wave (with no negative deflection).

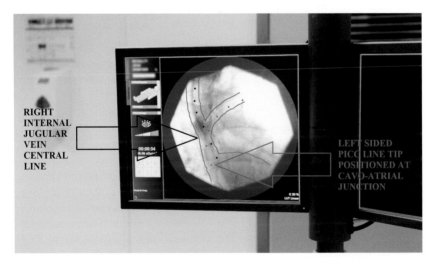

Figure 9.17 This patient was receiving TPN via a right internal jugular vein central line, which is visible on the x-ray marked out with black dots. The PICC line, which is marked out with red dots, is coming across the screen from the left side with the tip lying at the cavo-atrial junction.

- *Drainage*. Attach the normal saline syringe to the end of the PICC line after removing the stylet and freely aspirate venous blood to confirm it is in the vein. You can also take blood for laboratory testing at this point if so desired.
- *Examination*. Again, use a push, pause (stop, start) flushing technique to ensure catheter patency. At this stage, you should be confident that the PICC line is in the right position and functioning properly. If you have used real-time ECG guidance/x-ray screening and are not confident that the PICC line is in the intended position, you can request a formal departmental chest x-ray.
- *Fixation*. Using sterile swabs, clean and dry the area around where you have inserted the midline. Apply the fixation device to the PICC line and the patient's arm.

In closing, you should label the PICC line, fill in the insertion documentation for the patient notes and clear the trolley and dispose of any sharps and clinical waste. Also, thank the patient, make sure he/she is okay, and answer any questions the patient may have. According to your own institutional guidelines, you might also consider heparinising the catheter lumens.

Tips & Tricks for PICC Line Insertion

- Once you have cut the PICC line to the desired length, re-advance the stylet to within 1 cm of the end of the line. This 1 cm of line that is floppy will make it easier for the PICC line tip to follow the venous path towards the right atrium.
- PICC lines are designed primarily for infusion of TPN and chemotherapy. This needs a high-flow venous conduit with thick venous walls. Therefore, the line has to be positioned centrally, i.e., in the lower third of the superior vena cava.
- If the PICC line tip enters the internal jugular vein, then all you need to do is withdraw the line and try again. Asking the patient to turn his/her head towards you and tuck the chin is a technique that should prevent jugular vein entry. Alternatively, an assistant can perform ultrasound scanning of the ipsilateral internal jugular vein and compress the vein under vision.
- It is recommended that a single lumen PICC line is used where possible. This is to reduce the risk of thrombosis related to larger lumen sized devices.

PART 3
VENOUS ACCESS
AFTERCARE/OVERVIEW

CHAPTER 10

CARE & MAINTENANCE OF VENOUS LINES

Following insertion of a midline or a PICC line, it is important that the line be managed correctly to avoid complications. The most common problems encountered post-insertion are infection, catheter occlusion and accidental removal. These three complications are generally avoidable if proper care and maintenance are instituted.

Infection

It is not possible to keep lines completely sterile, as total freedom from micro-organisms is an unrealistic goal in typical healthcare settings. However, keeping the lines clean and aseptic is certainly achievable. 'Clean' means removing excessive dirt or contamination from around the exit site, and 'asepsis' means keeping the lines free from pathogenic organisms. The following dressing regimens are therefore recommended:

- Aseptic Non Touch Technique (ANTT) should be used when accessing midline and PICC line access devices.
- The dressings used should be transparent to allow visual inspection of the exit site. They should also be self-adhesive so they can provide added stability.
- The dressing should be semi-permeable to protect the site from bacteria and liquid whilst allowing the skin to breathe.
- Dressings should be inspected daily.
- Dressings should be changed at least every week or sooner if no longer intact or if moisture is collecting underneath.
- If the patient has profuse sweating or the insertion site is bleeding/oozing, then a sterile gauze dressing can be used. However, this gauze dressing should be changed to a transparent dressing as soon as possible.

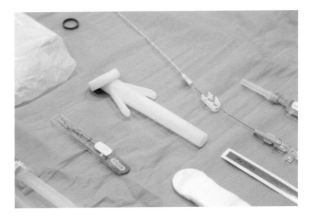

Figure 10.1 Alcohol cleaner.

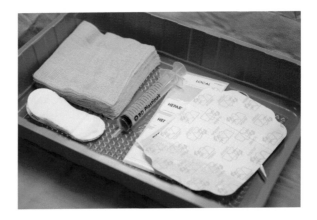

Figure 10.2 Sutureless securing device and overlying sticker.

- When changing dressings, the exit site should be cleaned with chlorhexidine 0.5% or 70% alcohol for at least 30 seconds (**Figure 10.1**).
- A stabilising device should be used to keep the line securely in place (**Figure 10.2**).

Maintaining Line Patency

Line occlusions are a common problem. There are a number of mechanical reasons why this may occur:

1. Intravenous (IV) tubing might be kinked or clamped.
2. Connections might be loose with air leaks.

3. The catheter itself may be kinked, twisted or misplaced.
4. Patient positioning may be the underlying cause.

Alternatively, the catheter may have become occluded by a blood clot. This can happen suddenly or gradually. In either case, it is often as a result of failure to flush the device. Another cause for occlusion of the catheter is because of fibrin deposition around the tip of the device. This is because of the body's reaction to a perceived irritant in the vascular system. The first sign of this fibrin sheath deposition is the inability to withdraw blood from the catheter – the vacuum created by the negative pressure of the aspirating syringe pulls this fibrin flap back against the opening of the catheter, and this prevents blood from entering the lumen. However, fluids can be delivered freely.

Flushing of catheters is therefore vitally important to maintain their patency:

- Catheters should be flushed with 0.9% normal saline.
- Devices should be flushed prior to and after each infusion.
- A turbulent flush should be used by using a 'push/pause' stop/start positive pressure technique. This will help remove debris from inside the catheter.
- Use a syringe that is no smaller than 10 mL for the flushing technique (this is to avoid excessive venous infusion pressures).
- Flushing should be performed weekly if the line is not in regular use (**Figure 10.3**).

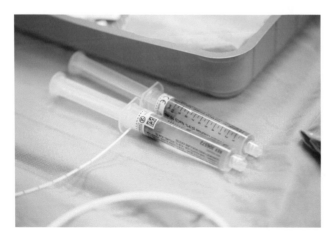

Figure 10.3 Normal saline syringes (10 mL each).

Line Stabilisation and Security

Once inserted, these lines are precious. It is therefore a priority to ensure that they are not accidentally pulled out. There are a number of different securing devices available, and each has its own individual merits. We recommend sutureless devices which are atraumatic compared to stitching the patient's skin. However, whatever your approach, of paramount importance is explaining to both the patient and the healthcare staff that they need to be very careful with the lines so as not to remove them inadvertently.

CHAPTER 11

COMPLICATIONS

In this chapter, we will review some theoretical 'worst-case' venous access complications. Although we have tried to make them 'realistic', they are not real cases and in our experience are extremely uncommon to encounter. We have chosen to focus on such challenging and difficult examples specifically because they illustrate the major principles that underpin both how to handle and also avoid such major complications. Indeed, by taking the lessons from these examples, we hope that you will never encounter such situations.

Example 1

You are a final-year medical student. You have been trained to insert midlines under supervision by one of the senior ward doctors. You have inserted three so far under direct supervision. The ward is quite busy and the senior doctor asks if you can insert a midline on an elderly patient who needs it for long-term antibiotics. Normally, this doctor would assist you, but he is called away to a medical emergency. You therefore decide to insert the midline on your own.

You wheel the patient into the treatment room at the bottom of the ward. It is very sunny outside but you do not know how to close the blinds. You set up your equipment and proceed. It is difficult to see the ultrasound image because of the sunlight. You proceed with needle cannulation and bright red blood freely flows from the end of the needle. You are confident that you have cannulated the basilic vein so you insert the guidewire and sheath. You then remove the inner sheath and guidewire and there is obvious pulsatile arterial bleeding. You immediately pull the whole sheath out and press on the area for 1 minute. Unfortunately, the whole puncture site rapidly swells and the patient experiences severe pain in his arm, which soon begins to turn a pale colour.

Diagnosis
- Brachial artery puncture
- Expanding haematoma

- +/− False aneurysm
- +/− Acutely ischaemic limb

Management

- Get help.
- Apply manual pressure over the puncture site for 10 minutes. The chances of successful occlusion of the brachial artery puncture site are improved by pressing directly down over the puncture site, with the artery being compressed against the underlying humerus bone. It is also helpful to have the patient's arm resting on a firmer surface (a soft pillow will make it more difficult to compress the arm downwards). Consider also using the ultrasound probe to press directly over the artery at the site of injury.
- Will need urgent vascular surgery assistance if there is expanding haematoma and/or loss of distal limb perfusion (i.e., cold hand, no pulses).

Factors Contributing to This Complication

- Inexperienced and unsupported trainee/student.
- Poor visualisation of ultrasound screen.

How to Avoid This Complication

- If you are performing an invasive procedure, have people close by within hearing distance in case you need to get help.
- Always have an assistant.
- If you are junior, inexperienced or a student, then don't perform invasive procedures without a senior present.
- Set the room and equipment up so it is working for you, not against you. In this case, the blinds should have been closed to block out the sun.

Example 2

You are a general surgery trainee. You have just learned how to insert PICC lines and have performed about five cases independently. You and your consultant have just performed an emergency Hartmann's procedure for a nasty diverticular perforation. The procedure was really difficult because of previous surgery and adhesions and took much longer than expected. Your consultant has just finished closing the abdomen and asks you to insert a PICC line for TPN post-operatively. The patient is still under a general anaesthetic. It is 3 a.m. You are very tired, haven't eaten or drunk anything for 4 hours and this is your fourth night shift in a row.

You are in a rush to complete the procedure. You puncture the patient's left basilic vein with the needle, insert the guidewire, and then proceed to insert the sheath over the wire. Unfortunately, as you are doing this, there is some commotion at the anaesthetic end of the table – the anaesthetist has told a joke and a few people start laughing. You lose concentration for a few seconds and when you look down, the wire has completely gone inside the sheath. The sheath is almost entirely within the patient's arm. You quickly pull the sheath back and remove it. The wire is hanging out of the skin by only a few millimetres. You try to grab it with your finger, but you have two layers of gloves on and can't grab it. Unfortunately, the wire disappears beneath the skin.

Diagnosis
- Guidewire lost into venous system

Management
- Do not release the tourniquet.
- Keep the patient in theatre under general anaesthesia.
- If such a situation arises and you haven't seen the guidewire disappear into the vein (i.e., it seems to have vanished), consider looking on the floor/around the patient to make sure it hasn't just dropped out accidentally.
- Don't attempt further manipulation or a surgical dissection to capture the guidewire. This is likely to force the guidewire further into the patient.
- Ask for anaesthetic support/cardiac monitoring to be set up in case the guidewire advances to the heart and causes arrhythmias
- Call for vascular surgery assistance.

Ultimately, if the wire is completely inside the venous system, interventional radiology will need to snare it out. If the wire tip is just under the skin but still out of the vein, it might be accessible by dissection of the skin just above and proximal to the puncture site; however, this is best performed by a vascular surgeon.

Factors Contributing to This Complication
- *Terrible combination*: fourth night shift, tired, hungry, thirsty, in a rush, theatre staff causing unnecessary distractions, double-gloving when trying to perform a delicate procedure.

How to Avoid This Complication

- The PICC line could have waited until tomorrow. In any case, you were not in a fit state to insert the line.
- Wear single gloves for delicate procedures.
- Always keep an eye on the guidewire, and if you have an assistant, have him/her hold onto it to stop this from happening.
- If you need to concentrate, request that other people in the room be quiet.

Example 3

You are an emergency medicine trainee in a busy tertiary hospital. It is 11 p.m. and a patient has been brought into the resuscitation bay by the ambulance crew. You have a 36-year-old intravenous drug user before you who is very well known to the department (he is a frequent attender and is known to sleep on the streets). According to his most recent discharge summary, he self-discharged from a medical ward last week after having a midline inserted for long-term intravenous antibiotics for infective endocarditis. He absconded from the ward with the midline in. Now he presents with a purple, blistered and grossly swollen left arm. The patient is profoundly unwell and in septic shock.

Diagnosis

- Necrotising fasciitis

Management

- SEPSIS 6 (blood cultures, check serum lactate level, high-flow oxygen, broad-spectrum intravenous antibiotics, catheterise and monitor fluid balance, intravenous fluids)
- Multi-disciplinary approach: Intensive care, anaesthetics, plastic surgery, vascular surgery
- Patient will require midline removal and radical debridement in theatre +/− upper limb amputation

Factors Contributing to This Complication

- Notoriously difficult patient cohort to manage.
- Self-discharges/long absences from wards common.
- Poor hygiene, issues with care and maintenance of line, and line abuse is not unusual.

How to Avoid This Complication

- Very difficult to avoid.
- This patient group commonly requires midlines/central lines for a variety of reasons, e.g., infective endocarditis, difficult access, infected groin pseudo-aneurysms, etc.
- A blanket statement of not inserting lines in this patient cohort is unrealistic.
- However, if they do require a line, then the patient must comply with the treating medical team. Misbehaviour, abuse of staff, non-compliance, long unexplained absences from the ward, and so on, are not to be tolerated. If these patients are not willing to behave responsibly and are likely to self-discharge, then frankly it is better to remove the line and treat with oral antibiotics.
- Be extremely cautious about self-administered outpatient parenteral antimicrobial therapy (S-OPAT) in this patient cohort.

Example 4

You are a medical trainee on-call in a busy tertiary hospital. You have been called down to review a very sick patient on a trauma ward. You turn up to find a young gentleman who has both his arms in plaster casts with a neck brace on. He was involved in a road traffic accident 12 days before and at that time sustained bilateral upper limb open humeral fractures and a cervical-spine fracture. He required a common femoral vein line for intravenous access. The line has been kept in because it was his only definitive form of venous access.

Now his right groin is slightly swollen and red around the line puncture site. He is spiking temperatures, has a blood pressure of 80/30 mmHg, a heart rate of 120, and very raised inflammatory markers. He looks flushed and sweaty and is warm to touch. His urine dip is normal, chest sounds clear on auscultation, and his abdomen is soft and non-tender. His arm wounds were reviewed the day before, and the nurse looking after him says the wounds were looking very healthy. He has had three bags of intravenous fluids, but his blood pressure continues to drop.

Diagnosis

- Septic shock due to infected femoral line

Management

- SEPSIS 6 (blood cultures, check serum lactate level, high-flow oxygen, broad-spectrum intravenous antibiotics, catheterise and monitor fluid balance, intravenous fluids)
- Urgent intensive care referral
- Remove line and send tip for culture

Factors Contributing to This Complication

- Lower limb venous access should be a last-resort option. In particular, the groin is a dirty area, and this is why the upper limb/neck is the preferred venous access routes in most patients.

How to Avoid This Complication

- Once a femoral line has served its purpose, remove it as soon as possible and consider other access options if available.
- Line care and maintenance is vitally important. If this line had been inspected and signs of infection identified earlier, the deterioration to septic shock might have been avoided.

Example 5

You are a senior anaesthetic trainee covering the emergency theatre in a small district general hospital. It is 3 a.m. Usually it is quiet overnight and you get to sleep. Your consultant is also at home sleeping. You have been woken up by the general surgeon on-call who says there is a sick 74-year-old patient with a gastric perforation who needs an emergency laparotomy. You go to see the patient, who is very high risk, and after discussing with your consultant, you both agree he needs an arterial line, central line and general anaesthetic. The consultant offers to come in, but as you are fairly senior, you say you are happy to manage the case on your own. You also want to impress your consultant by showing that you can handle such high-risk cases independently.

You have the patient in the anaesthetic room, which is very small. You are trying to insert the central line under ultrasound guidance, but it is so cluttered that your position is awkward and you feel very uncomfortable. The patient also has a very short fat neck and he has difficulty rotating his neck. You struggle to visualise the vein, as the ultrasound image is really dark. You cannot adjust the image because you are sterile and your assistant does not know how to adjust the settings. You struggle for a few minutes visualising the vein when the general surgery consultant enters the room and asks how long you are going to take. You feel flustered by his interruption and rush the procedure. There is a flash of pulsatile blood from your needle. You realise you have punctured the carotid artery. The patient starts talking nonsense and his face starts to droop. His arm also goes limp. Very soon he drops his conscious level.

Diagnosis
- Carotid artery puncture and stroke
- Possible carotid dissection/plaque rupture and distal embolization

Management
- Stop procedure, remove needle and apply manual pressure on neck
- ABCDE approach (Airway, Breathing, Circulation, Disability, Exposure and Examination)
- Call for help
- Ask your consultant to come in urgently
- Multi-disciplinary team management: Stroke, anaesthetics, general and vascular surgery, intensive care

Factors Contributing to This Complication
- No consultant support with very sick, high-risk and challenging patient.
- Room set-up poor and claustrophobic.
- Ultrasound settings sub-optimal.
- Inconsiderate behaviour from surgical team, who are putting you under pressure to rush.
- Late at night.

How to Avoid This Complication
- If it is an emergency case in the middle of the night with a high-risk patient and you are a trainee, no matter how senior you are, you will always benefit from senior support.
- Get your room and equipment set-up sorted before you start the procedure. Don't work in claustrophobic conditions.
- Have a sign outside the anaesthetic room saying 'Please do not interrupt when patient is being anaesthetised'.
- Never rush an invasive procedure, especially not when you are inserting a needle into the vicinity of major vascular structures.

Example 6

You are a middle-grade nephrology doctor. You are on the ward in the treatment room inserting a dialysis line on a patient with renal failure. This patient has had multiple lines before and failed fistulas. The patient has a slightly swollen arm on the side that you are inserting the line. You puncture the right internal jugular vein and insert the guidewire. It goes in relatively easily. You insert the sheath over the guidewire and encounter a considerable degree of resistance. The patient feels fine so you insert the sheath in fully. Suddenly, the patient experiences pain in his chest. He rapidly turns grey and clammy. He says he feels dizzy. You ask for help. A healthcare assistant rushes in. You get some observations which reveal a blood pressure of 60/40 mmHg and a heart rate of 140. Suddenly, the patient collapses on the floor in front of you.

Diagnosis
- Laceration of the right brachiocephalic vein communicating with the right pleural space
- Massive haemothorax

Management
- CRASH team alert
- Basic/advanced life support
- Will require cardiothoracic surgery intervention for definitive treatment

Factors Contributing to This Complication
- Failure to recognise clinical signs of central venous stenosis (arm swelling, and if you had examined patient's chest, you would have seen venous dilatation/collaterals).
- Complicated patient representing truly 'difficult' venous access.

How to Avoid This Complication
- Thorough history and examination is vital. Always ask about previous lines/surgery, etc.
- Pre-procedural ultrasound assessment of IJV may have shown that it did not compress easily, indicating central vein stenosis/obstruction.
- Complicated cases like these should be discussed in renal access multi-disciplinary team meetings and managed by specialists.

Example 7

You are a middle-grade anaesthetic trainee. You are fairly experienced; hence, your consultant has gone to sit in the theatre coffee room whilst you insert a central line on a very thin elderly patient prior to an elective laparotomy for a bowel cancer. The patient is needle phobic and extremely anxious. You insert a very small amount of local anaesthetic under the skin, which the patient tolerates. You go to insert the main needle, aiming for the internal jugular vein. It penetrates only a few millimetres when all of a sudden the patient leaps forwards and screams in pain. The needle accidentally inserts straight down beyond the patient's clavicle. As the patient writhes about in pain, the needle gets ripped out. The patient recovers and seems okay. However, over the next few minutes, she develops increasing shortness of breath. She rapidly deteriorates in front of you. Her trachea is deviated to one side and her entire lung field has no breath sounds.

Diagnosis
- Tension pneumothorax

Management
- Call for help
- Get senior assistance.
- Immediate needle decompression 2nd intercostal space mid-clavicular line
- Chest drain insertion

Factors Contributing to This Complication
- Needle-phobic patient making procedure higher risk.
- Very thin patient making it easier to puncture lung pleura.
- Inadequate amount of local anaesthetic.

How to Avoid This Complication
- If the patient understands the procedure, trusts the clinician, and feels comfortable, then he/she is likely to tolerate the procedure very well. Therefore, make a special effort to explain to the patient what you are doing, reassure him/her that everything is okay, make sure he/she is comfortable, and give plenty of local anaesthetic. Remember: If the patient is happy, the clinician is happy.

Example 8

You are a general surgery trainee. You have been asked by your consultant to insert a PICC line in a frail elderly gentleman who has multiple co-morbidities. This patient has recently had a bowel resection for a cancer and currently has an ileus. Your consultant explains that he needs the PICC line for total parenteral nutrition. You don't go to review the patient on the ward because your consultant has done so and you trust that everything will be okay. The theatre team send for the patient.

When the patient arrives, he is extremely aggressive and confused. He almost needs to be held down to insert the line. The line is a real struggle to insert, but eventually you get it in because you have a good theatre assistant who calms the patient and distracts him. Once you have confirmed the line position on x-ray and stuck the line down, you turn around to go and fill in the paperwork.

Immediately there is a loud crash and a scream. You turn around to see the patient on the floor beside the bed. There is blood pouring out onto the floor from where the PICC line has got caught on the bedrail and been ripped out. The patient has a nasty wound in his left arm where the thin skin has been torn, and his biceps muscle is visible underneath. You help lift the patient back up onto the bed, and he is screaming in pain. He is pointing to his left hip. His left leg is shortened and externally rotated. You ask the radiographer to do a quick x-ray of his left hip, which confirms a hip fracture.

Diagnosis

- Left neck of femur fracture
- PICC line accidental removal
- Soft tissue injury

Management

- ABCDE approach (Airway, Breathing, Circulation, Disability, Exposure and Examination)
- Analgesia
- Bandage arm
- Orthopaedic and plastic surgery referral

Factors Contributing to This Complication

- Not seeing the patient yourself prior to the procedure. If you had done this, you would have found out how unsuitable this patient was for a PICC line. He was very confused and aggressive on the ward and had already fallen out of bed three times this week and required constant supervision. He was also on warfarin and had an international normalised ratio (INR) level of 4.0.

How to Avoid This Complication

- Always go and see the patient.
- **You** decide if the PICC line is indicated or not. If the risks outweigh the benefits, then don't proceed.
- Have situational awareness and know what is going on around you. If you had gone to the ward and spoken to the nurses about this patient, you would have known he was at high risk for falling out of bed. Don't have tunnel vision and only be thinking about inserting the line. Think of the bigger picture.

Example 9

You are a senior medical trainee. You have been requested to insert a midline in an 18-year-old female patient because she is very difficult to cannulate and requires 3 days of intravenous antibiotics for cellulitis. The patient is systemically well, but your juniors are struggling to cannulate her forearms and she is complaining about all the bruising and pain. The midline insertion is straightforward and the patient thanks you. However, you did not formally consent her because you view midline insertion as a routine minor procedure no different than a cannula insertion.

You go on holiday the following day for 1 week. You return to work and your consultant asks to see you in private. You go into her office and she explains to you that whilst you have been abroad this patient had a pulmonary embolism and the family have put in a formal complaint. They have complained that the patient was never told about the risks of a pulmonary embolism. The consultant also informs you that the patient was on the oral contraceptive pill, there is a family history of venous thromboembolism, and the patient was not prescribed appropriate venous thromboembolic prophylaxis whilst in hospital.

Diagnosis

- Pulmonary embolism following midline line insertion

Management

- Remove line
- Anticoagulation
- Comply with whatever investigations take place surrounding the incident
- Learn from your mistakes

Factors Contributing to This Complication

- Inappropriate insertion of midline in patient with multiple risk factors for venous thromboembolism.

How to Avoid This Complication

- Don't insert long lines for 3 days of intravenous access. An ultrasound-guided cannula would have been suitable in this context.
- Consent patients for midlines and PICC lines and mention the key risks and possible alternatives. If you had done this properly, you would have probably not inserted a midline in the first place.
- History and examination is important so you know about the patient and relevant medical history.

Example 10

You are a general surgery trainee. You are on your lunch break when your phone rings. It is the emergency theatre coordinator. She informs you that there is a PICC line on the emergency theatre list that has been requested by one of your team. The emergency list has a free slot. They want to send for the patient. You say you are free so please send for the patient. You will see and consent the patient in the anaesthetic room.

When the patient arrives, you explain the PICC line procedure and risks and get him to sign the consent form. The patient agrees that he needs a line for feeding but seems very confused about the PICC line indication, but you carry on anyway. As the patient is wheeled into theatre, the patient asks for clarification about the PICC line again, and specifically asks why he needs it. You explain things again. You then insert the line without complication. One hour later, your consultant rings you to say you inserted the PICC line in the wrong patient and this is a 'serious incident' that will have to be investigated.

Diagnosis

- PICC line insertion in wrong patient

Management

- Apologise to patient
- Comply with serious incident investigation
- Learn from your mistakes

Factors Contributing to This Complication

- In this example, the PICC line was requested on the wrong patient by a junior member of the referring team. It had also been booked in the emergency theatre incorrectly by the referring team. You incorrectly assumed the patient had been vetted and approved by one of your trusted colleagues.

How to Avoid This Complication

- Always go and see the patient on the ward beforehand, and confirm for yourself that the line is required. Also, book the patient for the midline/PICC line yourself. Don't rely upon 'other people', even trusted colleagues, as ultimately it is *you* who are responsible if you are performing the procedure.
- Listen to the patient – In this case, the patient knew he needed a 'line' for feeding but actually had been told he needed a nasogastric tube for feeding, and the PICC line was not what he had expected. This was the first clue something was amiss. The actual PICC line was meant for the patient next door!
- Trust your instincts, and if something doesn't feel right, then don't proceed.

Example 11

You are an orthopaedic trainee. You are inserting a midline in a patient who has recently had a washout of a septic knee joint (who requires long-term intravenous antibiotics). The patient has some breathing difficulties because of a post-operative pneumonia. He is sitting up slightly and is gasping for breath throughout the procedure. The patient is also quite dehydrated and has an acute kidney injury. You have cannulated the basilic vein and the sheath is fully inside the patient's arm. You go to remove the inner sheath and guidewire when you suddenly hear a sucking sound. The patient deteriorates rapidly in front of you. He is complaining of chest pain and worsening dyspnoea. He becomes very tachycardic and hypotensive and his conscious level drops.

Diagnosis

- Air embolism

Management

- ABCDE approach (Airway, Breathing, Circulation, Disability, Exposure and Examination)
- Call for help
- Lie patient in left lateral position
- Administer 100% oxygen
- Terminate procedure
- Senior medical/anaesthetic support

Factors Contributing to This Complication

- Poorly hydrated patient
- Breathless and gasping patient
- Patient sitting up during procedure

These factors increase the likelihood that air can be sucked into the central veins, resulting in right ventricular dysfunction and pulmonary injury.

How to Avoid This Complication

- Valsalva manoeuvre increases pressure in the thoracic cavity.
- Ensure patients are adequately hydrated prior to line insertion.
- Make sure all lines/sheaths are flushed with normal saline.
- Avoid sitting patients up during line insertions.

How to Deal with a Complication

1. *Pre-empt with a formal consent process.* Although we do not believe written consent is necessary for a peripheral cannula insertion, for all the other venous access procedures in this book, we strongly recommend a formal written consent process. When you consent, you make it clear to both yourself and the patient what the common and relevant risks are. For most venous access techniques we discuss in this book, these are the risks we routinely mention: neurovascular injury,

bleeding, bruising/swelling, DVT/PE, infection, air embolism and line placement problems.

2. *Look & listen.* Use your eyes and ears. Pick up clues from what the patient tells and shows you. This might warn you of a pending complication. For example, a patient may tell you that she is on the oral contraceptive pill and her mother has had a pulmonary embolism. This should obviously warn you that she is at risk of a DVT. Another patient may tell you he has a severe needle phobia, and this should warn you that the patient may not lie still during the procedure. Another patient may tell you she has previously had a tunnelled line at another hospital and the doctor struggled to get the line in, and this may indicate a central venous stenosis. During the procedure itself, if the patient tells you that it is a lot more painful than he/she expected or their haemodynamic parameters alter, then these are again warning signs that something might have gone wrong. Don't ignore these warnings.

3. *Recognise and treat complications early on with simple effective measures.* As soon as you suspect something is not right, then stop what you are doing. Recognise quickly what the complication is and act with simple measures to help the situation. Don't just carry on, as this will likely make things worse. For example, if you have punctured an artery accidentally with the needle, then withdraw the needle and apply pressure. If you have caused a pneumothorax, then give the patient oxygen and ask for a chest x-ray and/or the chest drain set. If the patient has a cardiac arrest, then start chest compressions and call for the arrest team. Keep things simple.

4. *Ask for help.* Don't struggle on your own. If you are in trouble, then an extra pair of hands will always be beneficial. Your initial helper does not have to be a specialist. It doesn't take a skilled person to grab the crash trolley, do chest compressions, press over an artery with a swab, put on an oxygen mask, etc.

5. *Get specialist assistance if required.* If you encounter a complication that requires a specialist to deal with it, then get that specialist's help as soon as possible. For example, if you have caused a vascular injury, then call vascular surgery. If there is an arrthymia during a central line insertion, then ask for medical/cardiology/anaesthetic assistance. No one expects you to fix every complication on your own, but you are expected to get help from the right people. Also remember that it is better to be safe than sorry. If the specialist arrives and they are not required, then it might be a bit embarrassing. However, if you don't call the specialist until 4 days later when the patient's situation is beyond repair, then you will feel immensely worse.

6. *Be a professional.* Be polite, caring and considerate. Look presentable. Take pride in your work and do a good job. Don't laugh and joke and sing along to the radio whilst you are performing the procedure. Don't answer your phone when the patient is asking you questions. If you look and behave like a professional, then if and when you encounter a complication, the patient is more likely to be understanding and look upon you favourably.

7. *Handle the complication positively.* Everyone encounters complications. Sometimes you have made obvious mistakes, and other times it genuinely wasn't your fault. Don't blame yourself for everything, but likewise don't blame everyone and everything around you. Learn from the complication so it doesn't happen again. Apologise for whatever has occurred, but remember an apology does not mean you are accepting the blame. Comply with any investigations that take place surrounding the event. Get senior support and advice. Don't allow yourself to become cynical, negative, overly critical and depressed. Don't run away for fear of facing complications again. If you have fallen off your bike, yes, it hurts and it might be embarrassing, but get back on and keep cycling.

CHAPTER 12

SINGLE BEST ANSWER ASSESSMENT

Questions	111
Answers	118

Questions

Question 1

A 48-year-old female with recurrent metastatic breast cancer requires 6 months of chemotherapy. The plan is for her to have infusions around once a week on an outpatient basis. The patient has an active lifestyle and enjoys swimming regularly. She is right handed and has previously had a right mastectomy and axillary node clearance. On examination, she has good peripheral veins in both arms, although the right arm is slightly swollen compared to the left. She has normal basilic and brachial veins bilaterally and normal internal jugular veins on both sides.

The optimal choice for venous access in this patient is:

- A. PICC line via the right arm.
- B. Midline via the left arm.
- C. Tunnelled catheter via the left arm.
- D. Totally implanted port via the left internal jugular vein.
- E. Central non-tunnelled line via the right internal jugular vein.

Question 2

A 21-year-old female is admitted to the emergency department with sudden-onset right iliac fossa pain and collapse at home. The patient informs you that she is sexually active and not on any form of contraception currently. Her urine pregnancy test is positive. On examination, she has a heart rate of 120 with a blood pressure of 80/50 mmHg. She is peripherally shut down and you cannot easily find any veins in the hands or forearms. With a tourniquet, you identify reasonable veins in the antecubital fossae.

The optimal choice for venous access in this patient is:

- A. Blue cannula in left antecubital fossa.
- B. Orange/grey/green cannulas in both antecubital fossae.

   C. Midline via long saphenous vein.
   D. PICC line via left basilic vein.
   E. Central line via femoral vein in either groin.

Question 3

A 36-year-old male is referred to the acute medical assessment by his community doctor, who saw him this morning in clinic. He is complaining of shortness of breath on exertion and a productive cough. The patient informs you that he walked to the hospital as he lives only 15 minutes away. He appears systemically well and his oxygen saturations at rest are normal. On auscultation of his chest, you can hear some crepitations and bronchial breathing in the right lung base. His inflammatory markers are slightly raised. The patient has very good veins in both hands and forearms even without a tourniquet applied. He is right handed.

The optimal choice for venous access in this patient is:

   A. Blue cannula via right hand.
   B. Pink cannula via left antecubital fossa.
   C. Central line via left internal jugular vein.
   D. Venous access not required – oral antibiotics for mild community-acquired pneumonia will suffice.
   E. Orange cannula via right hand.

Question 4

A 79-year-old female on the elderly care ward is being treated for urinary sepsis and acute kidney injury. She has multiple comorbidities and is very frail. She also has poor oral intake and appears very dehydrated. She has very feeble veins in the back of her hands and forearms. She already has numerous bruises in both arms from venepuncture and failed cannulation attempts. Ultrasound assessment reveals healthy basilic veins bilaterally and normal internal jugular veins on both sides of her neck. Currently she requires intravenous antibiotics and fluids. She is expected to be in hospital for over 1 week.

The optimal choice for venous access in this patient is:

   A. Multiple blue or pink cannulas in either arm for the duration of her hospital stay.
   B. Central line.
   C. PICC line.
   D. Midline.
   E. Tunnelled catheter.

Question 5

A 30-year-old male is rushed into the emergency department following a high-speed road traffic accident. The patient, who was cycling to work on his bicycle, has been run over by a lorry. His left arm has been amputated at the level of the elbow and a tourniquet is above this level. Both his legs are grossly mangled and deformed to the level of his knees where the lorry wheels have crushed them. He is complaining of severe abdominal and chest pain. He is in grade 4 haemorrhagic shock. Currently, he only has a pink cannula inserted in his right wrist.

The optimal choice for venous access in this patient is:

A. Orange cannula via long saphenous vein at ankle level.
B. Grey cannula via back of right hand.
C. Tunnelled catheter via internal jugular vein.
D. Large-bore cannula via right antecubital fossa +/− internal jugular vein central line or femoral vein central line +/− intraosseous access.
E. Midline via right basilic vein.

Question 6

A 30-year-old female intravenous drug abuser is admitted to the cardiology ward with infective endocarditis. The patient requires 6 weeks of intravenous antibiotics. She has very poor venous access in the hands and forearms. She tells you that she has had three midlines in the left arm before and also DVTs in the left arm. Ultrasound scanning reveals occluded left basilic, brachial and cephalic veins, although on the right side they are healthy. Her internal jugular veins appear normal.

The optimal choice for venous access in this patient is:

A. Central line.
B. Tunnelled catheter.
C. Totally implanted port.
D. Midline via right arm.
E. PICC line via left arm.

Question 7

A 69-year-old gentleman is on the vascular surgery ward following an elective open AAA repair. His renal function has deteriorated slightly postoperatively and requires maintenance intravenous fluids for the next 24–48 hours. He has good veins in both his hands and forearms. Ultrasound assessment reveals healthy basilic veins in both upper arms and decent internal jugular veins. The patient is left handed.

The optimal choice for venous access in this patient is:

    A.   Green cannula in left antecubital fossa.
    B.   Pink cannula back of right hand.
    C.   Midline via left basilic vein.
    D.   PICC line via right basilic vein.
    E.   Central line via right internal jugular vein.

Question 8

A morbidly obese patient with decompensated heart failure is admitted to the cardiology ward with worsening shortness of breath. She is hypoxic and gasping for breath. She is finding it very difficult to lie down flat and demands that she be sat up. Her chest x-ray shows bilateral large pleural effusions with significant pulmonary oedema. Both her legs and forearms are oedematous. She requires urgent intravenous diuretic treatment. Her arms are so swollen that you cannot identify any veins in either arm despite using a tourniquet. Ultrasound assessment reveals an accessible cephalic vein in the mid forearm on both sides. She also has decent basilic/brachial veins in both upper arms.

The optimal choice for venous access in this patient is:

    A.   Central line.
    B.   Midline.
    C.   Tunnelled catheter.
    D.   Ultrasound-guided pink cannula via cephalic vein in either forearm.
    E.   Ultrasound-guided orange cannula via veins in back of hand.

Question 9

A 65-year-old female is on the orthopaedic ward following a washout of a left knee septic arthritis. She requires long-term intravenous antibiotics. She has previously had a nasty left clavicle fracture which was managed conservatively. Her left arm is more swollen than the right and she has prominent venous dilatation around her left upper chest wall and axillary region. On review of a chest x-ray performed a few months ago, you can see that the left clavicle has healed in a very deformed position. Ultrasound assessment reveals a healthy basilic vein on the right side. On the left side, the basilic vein appears much larger than the right and is slightly more difficult to compress. Her internal jugular veins appear normal.

The optimal choice for venous access in this patient is:

    A.   Tunnelled catheter via left subclavian vein.
    B.   Tunnelled catheter via right subclavian or internal jugular vein.

C. PICC line via right basilic vein.
D. Midline via right basilic vein.
E. Midline via left basilic vein.

Question 10

A 69-year-old diabetic female is on the neurosurgical ward following surgical treatment for lumbar vertebral discitis/osteomyelitis. She requires 6 weeks of intravenous antibiotics. She has previously had a left-sided radical neck dissection for a maxillofacial cancer 6 years ago. During this illness 6 years ago, she also had a PICC line inserted via the right arm for total parenteral nutrition and chemotherapy, which was unfortunately complicated by a right arm DVT. Ultrasound assessment reveals an occluded right basilic vein; however, the left basilic vein appears healthy. The internal jugular veins appear normal on both sides.

The optimal choice for venous access in this patient is:

A. Tunnelled catheter via left internal jugular vein.
B. Tunnelled catheter via right subclavian vein.
C. PICC line via left basilic vein.
D. Midline via left basilic vein.
E. Totally implanted port via left internal jugular vein.

Question 11

A 32-year-old female had a left-arm midline inserted 1 day ago for long-term intravenous antibiotics as an outpatient. She is on the oral contraceptive pill. She presents to the acute medical assessment unit with a swollen left arm. She is systemically well and apyrexial. The exit site of the midline looks normal with no signs of infection.

The appropriate course of action for this patient is:

A. Reassure the patient that this is normal and discharge her home.
B. Remove the midline immediately and request a new midline.
C. Anticoagulate and refer the patient for an urgent DVT scan.
D. Remove the midline and fully anticoagulate her for 6 months.
E. Request urgent thrombolysis.

Question 12

A patient is on a general surgery ward 5 days following an elective large bowel resection and stoma formation. The patient has a central line *in situ* which was inserted at the time of the operation. At the moment, the central line is not being used for treatment, but the ward doctors are aspirating blood from it daily to check the patient's blood results. The patient starts spiking temperatures, and he is showing signs of sepsis. There is no other obvious source of sepsis (abdomen is soft and nontender, stoma is functioning, chest is clear on auscultation, urine dip is negative).

The appropriate course of action for this patient is:

A. Request an urgent CT scan of his abdomen to see if the abdomen is the cause for his sepsis.

B. Commence him on oral antibiotics for sepsis of unknown origin.

C. Reassure the patient that a few temperature spikes postoperatively are normal.

D. Remove the central line and send the tip for culture. Commence him on appropriate intravenous antibiotics via a cannula in his hand/forearm.

E. Commence him on intravenous antibiotics via the central line.

Question 13

You are inserting a midline into a 63-year-old diabetic gentleman who needs long-term intravenous antibiotics for osteomyelitis of his heel. You attempt to cannulate the left basilic vein but struggle to gain access because the patient finds externally rotating his shoulder difficult (he has shoulder osteoarthritis). You puncture the vein and try to insert the guidewire but it will not advance. You attempt to puncture the vein further up the arm but encounter similar difficulties. On the ultrasound screen, you can see there is a large haematoma around the vein, and the vein has now gone into spasm and is very small. The brachial vein is very small and lying almost underneath the brachial artery, and you are worried if you try to cannulate it you might injure the artery.

The appropriate course of action for this patient is:

A. Have a third attempt at trying to cannulate the left basilic vein.

B. Attempt to cannulate the left brachial vein.

C. Stop the procedure and explain to the patient that he is not suitable for a midline and will require a Hickman line instead.

D. Attempt to insert a PICC line via the right arm.

E. Attempt to insert a midline via the right arm.

Question 14

You are inserting a PICC line into a patient via the left arm. You have failed to cannulate the basilic vein because it is very small and has now gone into spasm. The patient's left brachial vein appeared suitable, and you tried to cannulate it. As you advance the needle into the brachial vein, there is a jet of pulsatile red blood that shoots out of the back of the needle. You realise you have punctured the brachial artery.

The appropriate course of action for this patient is:

A. Insert the guidewire and sheath and call for vascular surgery assistance.
B. Remove the needle and using a swab apply pressure over the artery for 10 minutes.
C. Remove the needle and attempt to insert a midline on the right side.
D. Remove the needle and apply pressure over the artery for 30 seconds. Then re-attempt puncturing the brachial vein on the same side.
E. Remove the needle, reassure the patient, and try to cannulate the left cephalic vein.

Question 15

You are requested to insert a midline into a 99-year-old demented woman on an elderly care ward. The referral states that the patient needs maintenance intravenous fluids and a blood transfusion. She has apparently ripped out six cannulas in the past 2 days and the referring team are obviously struggling with intravenous access. You go to assess the patient on the ward. She is being closely monitored by a healthcare assistant because she has fallen out of bed three times this week. The bedrails are currently up and cushioned by numerous pillows. You go to examine her arms and see that they are extensively bruised. She has virtually no suitable veins for cannulation. You try to scan her upper arms to assess her basilic veins but the patient violently pushes you away. You notice the patient is very dehydrated and offer her a glass of water which she happily drinks. On checking the patient's blood results, you note she has deranged clotting because of warfarin treatment. Her full blood count also shows that she has mild anaemia (haemoglobin is 88). Her inflammatory markers are normal.

The appropriate course of action for this patient is:

A. Attempt a midline insertion via either basilic vein.
B. Encourage the patient to drink plenty of water and recommend that her anaemia be treated with oral iron tablets.
C. Explore her ankles to see if you can cannulate her long saphenous vein.
D. Recommend that the patient have a central line inserted.
E. Attempt an ultrasound cannula in either arm.

Answers

Question 1 = D. Totally implanted port via the left internal jugular vein.

The port is totally implantable and should therefore allow the patient to continue her active lifestyle normally. The long-term infrequent infusions of chemotherapy on an outpatient basis also make the port a very attractive option. If the chemotherapy was needed at more frequent intervals (i.e., multiple infusions per week) and the patient did not mind having an exterior line visible, then a tunnelled catheter or PICC line would potentially be more suitable. Of note, chemotherapy has to be delivered via central veins, making midlines unsuitable for chemotherapy.

Question 2 = B. Orange/grey/green cannulas in both antecubital fossae.

This patient has a ruptured ectopic pregnancy and is in haemorrhagic shock. She needs urgent short large-bore intravenous access via both antecubital fossa. This will allow her to have rapid infusion of intravenous fluids and blood products on her way to the operating theatre.

Question 3 = D. Venous access not required – oral antibiotics for mild community-acquired pneumonia will suffice.

This young gentleman does not warrant hospital admission nor treatment with intravenous antibiotics. He has a mild community-acquired pneumonia which can be managed with oral antibiotics at home. If he did require hospital admission for intravenous antibiotics, a blue/pink cannula in the dorsum of the hand/forearm would be recommended.

Question 4 = D. Midline.

This frail elderly woman will likely be in hospital for a while and will no doubt require intravenous access for various reasons throughout her stay. She has poor peripheral access and is already suffering by way of repeated cannulation attempts. A single definitive midline can be inserted via either of her suitable basilic veins.

Question 5 = D. Large-bore cannula via right antecubital fossa +/− internal jugular vein central line or femoral vein central line +/− intraosseous access.

This major trauma patient has life-threatening haemorrhagic shock. He requires immediate large-bore intravenous access so that fluids and blood products can be given immediately for resuscitation. Due to being run over by the lorry, his left arm and both legs below the level of the knees are not suitable for vascular access. His neck, right arm and both groins are therefore available for venous access (similarly, intraosseous access should also be considered).

Question 6 = D. Midline via right arm.

This patient requires long-term intravenous antibiotics. The left arm is clearly not suitable given the occluded veins in the upper arm. A midline via the right arm would enable long-term intravenous antibiotics and carries fewer risks than central venous access. If a midline were not possible, then a tunnelled catheter would be the next option to consider.

Question 7 = B. Pink cannula back of right hand.

With excellent veins in both his arms, a pink cannula should suffice for short-term intravenous fluid therapy.

Question 8 = D. Ultrasound-guided pink cannula via cephalic vein in either forearm.

This patient has oedematous arms and requires urgent diuretic therapy for decompensated cardiac failure. An ultrasound-guided pink cannula that can target either forearm cephalic vein would seem ideal. A midline would be another consideration, but in this context, the patient would not be able to lie down flat, and this would make access extremely difficult. In such a patient, however, a central line may likely be needed for ongoing definitive management, e.g., fluid management/inotropic support, etc.

Question 9 = D. Midline via right basilic vein.

For long-term intravenous antibiotic treatment, a midline would be the ideal treatment. However, given the clinical information, it seems as if the previous clavicle fracture has caused some damage to the left subclavian vein. The swelling of the arm, venous dilatation around the upper arm and chest, and difficulty compressing the left basilic vein are all pointing towards a subclavian/axillary vein stenosis/obstruction. Therefore, a right-sided midline seems most appropriate.

Question 10 = D. Midline via left basilic vein.

This patient is fairly complicated. The radical neck dissection makes central vein access potentially difficult from the left side. The right-sided DVT and occluded veins make right-sided upper arm access impossible. For long-term intravenous antibiotics, a midline would suffice and therefore should be attempted from the left side. If this does not work, then a tunnelled catheter via the left subclavian vein can be considered.

Question 11 = C. Anticoagulate and refer the patient for an urgent DVT scan.

At the moment, the patient is systemically well and has a swollen left arm. There may be no sinister underlying pathology and she may just require reassurance. However, a swollen arm following a midline insertion in the context of oral contraceptive pill use should alert you to the possibility of a DVT. The patient can be anticoagulated and referred for an urgent DVT scan. If there is no DVT, the anticoagulation can be ceased, and the patient can be reassured and discharged. If there is a DVT, the midline will have to be removed and the patient should continue with anticoagulation.

Question 12 = D. Remove the central line and send the tip for culture. Commence him on appropriate intravenous antibiotics via a cannula in his hand/forearm.

In this case, the central line has been left *in situ* without sufficient justification. A central line can be used to take blood, but if this is the only reason for keeping it, then the benefits do not outweigh the risks. It looks like the patient has line sepsis; therefore, the line should be removed, the tip sent for culture, and the patient treated with appropriate intravenous antibiotics via a cannula in either arm.

Question 13 = E. Attempt to insert a midline via the right arm.

Given his shoulder arthritis, access for a left-sided midline is clearly very difficult. You are struggling, and proceeding further on this left side seems risky. At this point, it would be best to apologise to the patient and explain that access from the left side is not ideal. You should attempt to insert a midline from the right side, which one hopes will be easier.

Question 14 = B. Remove the needle and using a swab apply pressure over the artery for 10 minutes.

Puncturing the brachial artery with the needle is not ideal, but it is not a total disaster. Remember that the brachial artery is frequently cannulated for the purpose of arterial access (e.g., arterial lines, upper limb angiograms, etc). If you puncture the artery, simply remove the needle and apply pressure over it for 10 minutes. Don't insert the guidewire and sheath, because this will only serve to create a bigger defect in the vessel wall. Once you have compressed the vessel, do not attempt further access on this arm. Definitely do not try to recannulate the brachial vein (there will likely be a haematoma around this area, which will make access more difficult). If there is no expanding haematoma and the perfusion to the hand is okay, then you can consider attempting a midline from the other side. If you have any concerns, ask for an urgent vascular surgery review.

Question 15 = B. Encourage the patient to drink plenty of water and recommend that her anaemia be treated with oral iron tablets.

In this situation, it is important to determine the patient's capacity (dementia doesn't mean incapacity). If the patient has capacity and is refusing the line, then you should not proceed. If the patient does not have capacity, then it would be sensible to refer back to the parent medical team for a discussion regarding what is in the patient's best interests. At the moment, it would be unwise to leap straight into a midline insertion. She is stable and therefore oral therapy can be recommended. Additionally, the patient fighting you off and the deranged clotting should veer you away from a midline insertion.

INDEX

Index

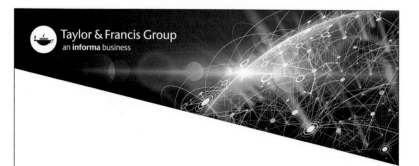

Taylor & Francis Group
an **informa** business

Taylor & Francis eBooks

www.taylorfrancis.com

A single destination for eBooks from Taylor & Francis
with increased functionality and an improved user
experience to meet the needs of our customers.

90,000+ eBooks of award-winning academic content in
Humanities, Social Science, Science, Technology, Engineering,
and Medical written by a global network of editors and authors.

TAYLOR & FRANCIS EBOOKS OFFERS:

A streamlined
experience for
our library
customers

A single point
of discovery
for all of our
eBook content

Improved
search and
discovery of
content at both
book and
chapter level

REQUEST A FREE TRIAL
support@taylorfrancis.com

 Routledge
Taylor & Francis Group

 CRC Press
Taylor & Francis Group